NEVER EVER GIVE UP!
SURVIVAL FROM CANCER!

By: Wang Zhen-Guo

Published and Distributed by:

Green & Gold International Exports
Rm. 307 Solmac Building
84 Dapitan cor. Banawe St.
Quezon City, Philippines
Tel. (632) 7810069, 4162951, 4158714
Fax (632) 4158715, 3616996
Email: info@cancerherbal.com
URL: http://www.cancerherbal.com

ISBN No. 962-542-013-4
ISBN No. 971-92063-1-4

Printed by
PHILIPPINE GRAPHIC ARTS, INC.
163 Tandang Sora Street, Caloocan City

Surprise to the World -
Cancer cured by Chinese Medicine

NEVER EVER GIVE UP!
SURVIVAL FROM CANCER!

**True stories from 50 people who have
successfully overcome cancer!**

Edited by: Wang Zhen-Guo
Medical Researcher, Ministry of Public Health, China
President, Anti-cancer Association of Jilin Province, China
President Chang Bai Shan Institute of Medicine, China

Revised Edition

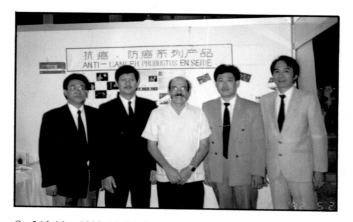

On 24th May 1992, Mr. Medina, the commercial & industrial leader in Mexico, visited President Wang Zhen Guo, the author of this book, in the Chinese Medicine Exhibition in Mexico

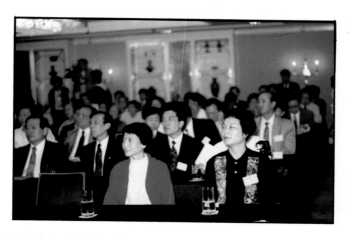

On 6th Nov 1992, President Wang made a speech in Island Shangri-la Hotel, Hong Kong

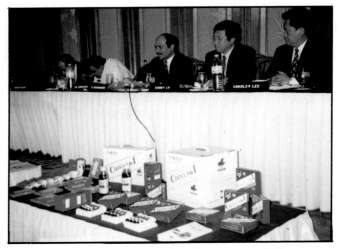

On 2nd Sep 1995, President Wang hosted a seminar in India

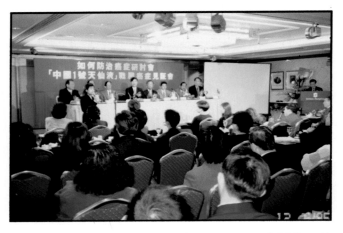

On 5th Dec 1995, Miss Wang Bi Yun from Taiwan attended "China No. 1 Tian Xian Liquid Fight against Cancer" Seminar in Island Shangri-la Hotel, Hong Kong

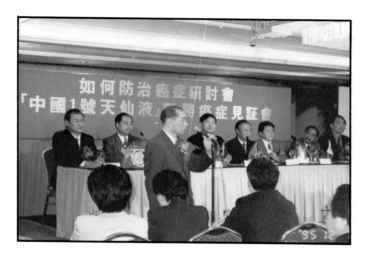

On 5th Dec 1995, Mr. Chen Yu Lin from Taiwan attended "China No. 1 Tian Xian Liquid Fight Against to Cancer" Seminar in Island Shangri-la, Hong Kong

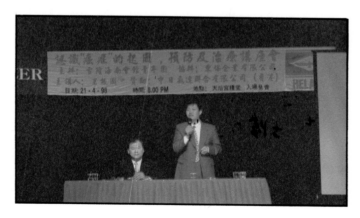

On 21st April 1998, President Wang made a speech in Malaysia

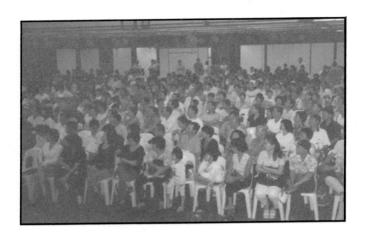

On 21st April 1998, President Wang made a speech in Sky Palace in Kuala Lumpur, Malaysia which attracted thousands of people.

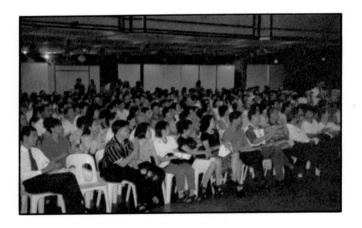

On 21st April 1998, thousands of people attended "The Truth of Tian Xian Liquid Seminar" in Sky Palace in Kuala Lumpur, Malaysia

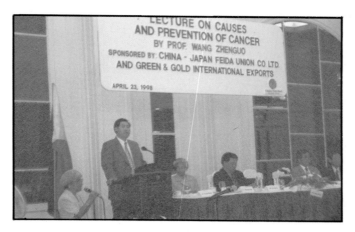

On 23rd April 1998, President Wang made a speech in Manila, Philippines

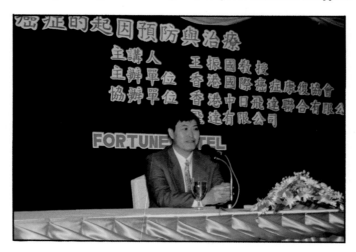

On 30th April 1998, President Wang made a speech in Bangkok, Thailand

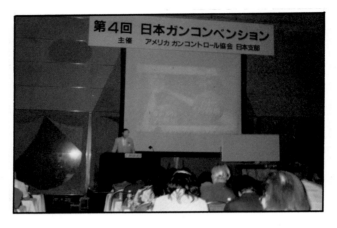

On 25th July 1998, the 4th Intl. Cancer Convention was hosted by the US
Cancer Control Association - Japan Branch in Tokyo, Japan. President
Wang was the only Chinese speaker of the Convention

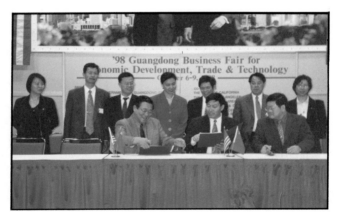

On 5th October 1998, the Chairman of China-Japan Feida Union Co. Ltd. -
Mr. Lu Chi Hui and President Wang signed an agreement in Los Angeles,
California, U.S.A. It made Chinese Medicine the focus of research on
biological technology in the following 10 years

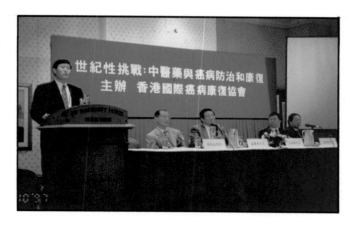

On 20th October 1998, President Wang made a report in the
"Seminar on Chinese Herbs and Cancer Prevention and Healing in
Regal Hotel, Hong Kong

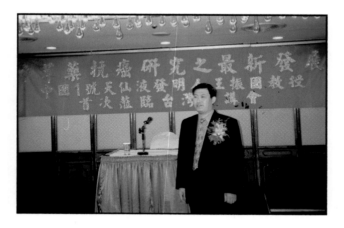

On 5th March 1999, President Wang first went to Taiwan. He made a
research report on "Prevent of Cancer with Chinese Herbs" in Lai Lai
Shangrila Hotel, Taipei

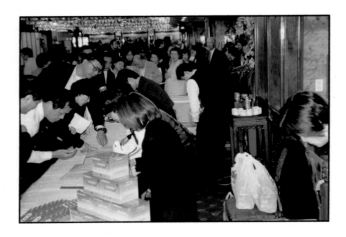

On 5th March 1999, President Wang made a speech in Lai Lai Shangri-la Hotel Taipei which attracted several hundreds of people.

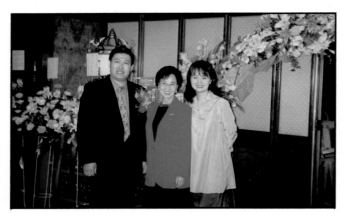

Famous Movie Star, Joan Deng and her mother took a photo with President Wang in Lai Lai Shangri-la Hotel, Taipei. They thanked "China No. 1 Tian Xian Liquid" for giving them a better health

INTRODUCTION

CANCER - A CURABLE DISEASE

BRINGING COURAGE AND JOY TO THOSE WHO
COMBAT CANCERS
"CHINA NO. 1 TIAN XIAN LIQUID WHICH BRINGS
IMPORTANT CONTRIBUTIONS TO OUR NATION IS WORTHY
OF PRAISE."

THIS IS what Chancellor JIANG Je-min said at the opening speech on his visit to the Changbai Mountain Institute, Tonghua City, Jilin Province and I felt exceptionally happy. In winter of 1991, I began my research study of China No.1 Tian Xian Liquid based on China No.1 Tian Xian Capsule.

When I was working on China No. 1 Tian Xian Capsule, I was glad to receive confirmation of its 'anti cancer effects' from clinical tests done at the Tianjin Pharmacology Institution. Later, my project was described as the 'most valuable research of the nation' and was included in the government's scientific and technological development program. It was classified as a national research project for leading hospitals and medical institutions throughout China.

In addition, a clinical report from the United States Anti cancer Center showed that the liquid has an 80% effective curative rate on cancer. So I continued to improve China No. 1 Tian Xian Capsule and the result was the world-renowned anti cancer treatment, China No. 1 Tian Xian Liquid

A new and improved treatment, China No.1 Tian Xian Liquid being extracted from natural herbs was born.

Because of the highest government ratings given nationwide clinical tests on the Liquid, Chancellor JIANG visited our institution located in the remote part of China.

According to World Health Organization (WHO), there are about 40 million people suffering from cancer worldwide. The number of new cancer patients is rapidly increasing at an estimated rate of 9 million per year. In China with a population of over 1.3 billion, there is an estimated 1.6 million new cancer cases each year. About 1 million or 14% of all deaths per year is said to be cancer related.

Japanese statistics states that 270,000 people died of cancer in 1996 (about 30% of its deaths) and estimates over 500,000 new cancer cases each year. In a medically advanced country like Japan and considering the low rate of cancer deaths compared to other countries, still the death rate is rising.

Even with our advanced knowledge of science, medicine and medical treatment, the panacea for cancer has not yet been developed. It is a fact that cancer is still the greatest enemy of the entire human kind.

In July of 1998, I was invited to a forum, "Cancer-The Possibility of Survival," which was conducted by the Japan Chapter of the US Cancer Control Association. I have been given the honor to deliver a speech at the Japanese International Cancer Convention. It was an occasion for medical researchers from around the world to share their experiences and achievements in developing cures against cancer. Details shall be elaborated in later chapters of this book. At the convention, I represented the Traditional Chinese Medicine and China No.1 Tian Xian Liquid became the center of attention.

The convention received wide coverage and attention in Japan. It is a good opportunity for cancer researchers to study the disease. We hope that a panacea for cancer will be developed in the near future and I will do our best to help the world fulfill the mission.

In the following pages of this book are detailed descriptions of the world-renowned China No.1 Tian Xian Liquid. Chapter 3 discussed everything about the medicine and Chapter 4 tells about the worldwide battle against cancer. Lastly, this book aims to spread the good news of China No. 1 Tian Xian Liquid to cancer patients everywhere and to promote the idea of 'cancer-a curable disease.' Lastly, to give hope to patient's to pursue a courageous fight in order to survive cancer and to enjoy life to the fullest.

Special thanks go to the chief editor, the members of the Japan Chapter of the International Cancer Rehabilitation Association and members of the Japan Medical and Treatment Planning.

Wang, Zhen - Guo
Researcher, China National Health Department
Director, Jilin Anti Cancer Association
Director, Changbai Mountain Pharmacology Institution
March, 1999

TABLE OF CONTENTS

1

TRIUMPHS OVER CANCER

THE AMAZING STORY OF NATURAL CHINESE MEDICINE

A REVOLUTION IN CANCER TREATMENT FOR THE FIRST TIME THE CHINESE GOVERNMENT REVEALS THE SECRETS OF CHINA NO. 1 TIAN XIAN LIQUID - A REVOLUTIONARY ANTICANCER CHINESE MEDICINE

CHAPTER
1

HOLISTIC HEALTH CARE:
A DEFINITION AND DISCUSSION

In 1926, the concept of "holistic" healthcare was first described as such by the South African philosopher Jan Christian Smuts. Virtually synonymous with the terms "wholistic, alternative," "biological," and "integral" medicine, holism was a manner of comprehending a living being as a whole organism, its systems greater and different from the sum of their parts.

Holistic medicine involves expanding our concept of healthcare to include the many personal, familial, social and environmental factors that promote health, prevent illness, and encourage healing. It encompasses and is at times undistinguished from humanistic, behavioral, and integral medicine, including an appreciation of patients as mental, emotional, social, spiritual as well as physical entities. It attempts to fully recognize the true causation of underlying triggering mechanisms through an attitude of viewing the human being from a total and whole perspective. Thus, the existence of an interdependent and inter influential functional relationship between man's organic behavior and his biological role in his environment should be the basis of any attempt to analyze, diagnose and treat the human being.

Man strives to maintain homogeneous conditions inside his body as well as compatible relationships with his environment. Starting from his cellular structure, his tissues, glands, and organ systems exist in a single body, bound by their physical structure and the interrelatedness and interdependence of their functions. The human being in turn responds to the various conditions in its environment. The totality of the human individual, his role in the ecosystem, his recognition and understanding of the fundamental law of nature, constitutes the basic precepts of holistic medicine.

Holistic medicine views the patient as an individual person, not as a symptom-bearing organism. It emphasizes the self-responsibility of the person for his or her health. Finally, it emphasizes the importance of mobilizing the individual's ability to preserve himself or herself, rather than depending on outside help to maintain health or manage disease. It respects the patient's capacity to play an active role in the healing of disease, and not just the passive recipient of healthcare. In the holistic approach, the patient is the best judge of himself, not the doctor. While the doctor is respected as a learned, experienced, professional consultant, the patient is not only a major partner as far as health matters concerning himself are concerned- he or she holds undisputed authority over health matters involving his or her well-being.

Holistic medicine makes judicious use of many standard diagnostic or therapeutic modalities in addition to its wide range of *materia medica* and alternative medical practices. Some alternative or traditional healing modalities enjoy the confidence and acceptance of orthodox medicine, while others, although used in holistic medicine, have yet to gain acceptance. These techniques will only be integrated into mainstream medical practice after more research on them is carried out and proof of their successful clinical application is provided.

26

Holistic medicine is made up of both conventional and alternative and traditional healing modalities. Some forms of alternative medicine, such as the manipulative therapies (massage, acupuncture, chiropractic) have become part of the conventional medical repertoire and are only considered alternative when claims for their value are greatly extended. Others are not currently in use among medical practitioners, but there would be no objections to their adoption would convincing proof of their value be presented. The fact that some procedures were derived from a discredited system does not conclusively indicate its lack of efficacy. It is generally accepted that acupuncture, particularly when combined with electrical stimulation, can modify the perception of pain.

The ideal practitioner of holistic medicine is a physician whose knowledge extends far beyond the limits of orthodox medicine. To effectively investigate his patient's problems, diagnose their conditions, offer an acceptable range of courses for treatment, and conduct definitive therapy requires a good working knowledge of alternative as well as allopathic medicine. Such a physician, for example, when faced with a case of chronic back pain, examines the patient physically, emotionally, nutritionally and mentally. Once a diagnosis has been made, he may select a therapeutic course of action based on acupuncture, herbal medicine, chiropractic, neurology, ayurveda, meditation, lifestyle modification and magnetic healing, or combinations of these modalities. The final therapeutic plan will depend not only on which modality or combination of modalities the doctor perceived to be best, but also on which course of action the patient has greatest confidence in and is most comfortable with.

The challenge of holistic medicine for health care workers, therefore, is formidable. The rewards to be gained, however, are well worth the effort. Modern science has demonstrated and acknowledges the interconnection between the psyche and the soma. Whether the explanation for the unity of mind and body be in the form of neural hormones of factors or energy fields, the fact is that such a relationship exists. Experienced physicians concede that, under certain situations, a patient can will himself back to good health, and that a strong attitude of determination has frequently spelled the difference between life or death. A medical system that integrates the advantages of the physical/scientific approach and the psychic/mental spiritual approach would be a powerful, versatile and potent system indeed. This is the basic strength of the holistic approach.

Holistic healthcare should not be synonymous with last-resort medical care. Many people believe that holistic medicine is less therapeutically potent than orthodox medicine, and that, since it utilizes 'alternative' medicine, it is to be used in situations where orthodox medicine has failed. As has been mentioned earlier, holistic medicine encompasses orthodox medicine, and is included in its scope. Furthermore, herbal medicine, acupuncture, chiropractic and many other therapeutic modalities have shown great promise, singly and in combination, as first-choice drugs or first line therapies for certain clinical conditions and settings. In its truest sense, therefore, holistic healthcare means quality, greater freedom of participation for the patient, and more options for the healthcare provider and consumer alike.

The trend towards holistic healthcare is not an isolated phenomenon. Many prominent practitioners, centers and learning institutions all over the world, particularly in the developed countries, have concentrated their energies on practicing, promoting and developing holistic medicine. These include the Bristol Health Clinic, which specializes in cancer, homeopathy, acupuncture and massage and was established with the help of Prince Charles; and the hospital for integrated healthcare, International Biologics, in Tijuana, Mexico which features laetrile therapy, fetal cell therapy, nutrition therapy and other varieties of alternative medicine.

Famous centers of learning, such as the Harvard Medical School, have integrated biological, traditional and alternative medicine courses into their curriculum. The University of the Philippines College of Medicine has also integrated the subject of values and orientation into its curriculum, while the De La Salle University School of Medicine has begun to offer acupuncture as part of medical training. The East Avenue Medical Center, on the other hand, became the first government hospital in the Philippines to offer a postgraduate course for physicians relevant to holistic healthcare. And the Capital University in Washington, the lone university in the United States that offers degrees on Holistic Medicine.

CHAPTER
2

THE CONCEPT OF INTEGRATED HEALTHCARE

WHY INTEGRATED HEALTHCARE?

A logical question to ask at this point is: Why should healthcare be integrated? What characteristics of the human being dictate that it should be so? The answer to this question is simple: because man is not a machine that may be disassembled system by system, piece by piece, aspect. One cannot take a symptom and treat it in isolation from the totality of the human being two displays or suffers from it. In short, this concept-that of the integrated Human Person (IHP)-presents a model of the human being that mixes man's physical, mental, emotional, intellectual and environmental properties in to one entity.

According to this model, any factor influencing one aspect of IHP actually affects the organism as a whole. Any modern effort at making health care relevant must take this model of the human being into consideration. The concept of integrated healthcare, therefore, was designed with the IHP in mind.

INTEGRATED HEALTHCARE IS PREVENTIVE MEDICINE

"An ounce of prevention is worth a pound of cure," goes an old adage. Preventive medicine deals with measures to protect the individual from disease and keep him in positive state of health. Environmental medicine is an important field which stresses the role that ecosystems play in the pathogenesis of disease. It is concerned with measures that can be taken to preserve the environment and maintain public health.

Hippocrates practiced medicine over 2,000 years ago and wrote the code of ethics. His teaching are strikingly relevant to the realities of the current healthcare system. He wrote about healing patients with food instead of drugs. He emphasized knowing the patient's personality type, diet and occupation as necessary determinants of the course of therapy to be given. He gave a detailed discussion of how food allergies can play an important role in genesis of disease.

Hippocrates said: "It is more important to know what kind of patient has a disease than what kind of disease a patient has. Your health cure will frequently depend more on your uniqueness than on the characteristic of your medical condition."

HEALTH DEFINED

In order to understand the concept of Integrated Healthcare, a definition of the term *Health* must first be agreed upon. The World Health Organization (WHO) defines health as a state of complete physical, mental and social well-being of an individual. This definition emphasizes the positive state of health, not merely the absence of disease.

To promote and maintain a positive state of health, the following basic elements are necessary: a supply of fresh air, sunlight, and safe, potable water, a balance diet, healthful shelter, adequate clothing, hygienic environmental sanitation; protection from communicable diseases, social and economic security, and a congenial socio-cultural atmosphere. In addition, an individual should have a regulated lifestyle with proper rest, relaxation and exercise.

CONCEPT OF HEALTH AND DISEASE

The world *health* is related etymologically to the Anglo-Saxon word from which are derived not only *healing,* but also *Holiness* and *wholeness.* Used to describe the state of living organism, health refers to the individual as a functional whole in which all necessary organic mechanism are present and acting cooperatively and harmoniously. Briefly, "Health is the state of being in which an individual does the best with the capacities he has, and act in ways that maximize his capacities."

Health is better defined as optimal functioning which means that each organ and organ system is functioning well and harmony with other organs and organ system. Together, their actions should form the life process of a single individual.

A human being is a dynamic or open system capable of maintaining homeostasis in relation to its environment by regulating the input and output of matter and energy in view of this concept of human functioning, we can see that health means not only the capacity of the organism to maintain itself in its environment but also its ability to create a function within itself.

According to the WHO, a person whose body processes are not functioning at their optimum level (and who, therefore, is not healthy) is not necessarily diseased or sick. It is possible for an organism to fall short of optimal functioning without being diseased or infirm. The lack of overt signs and symptoms of disease, therefore, does not necessarily indicate a state of health.

Two major concepts of disease exist, these being the ontological and the physiological models of disease. The ontological concept regards diseases as separate entities that can be classified like plants and animals. The physiological concept views disease as the disruption of the internal harmony of organic systems secondary to hypo (excessively weak) function or the hyper (excessively strong) function of an organ. Such a dysfunction renders the organism open to attack by external agents. If the organism were functioning properly, it would resist such an attack.

Physiologists correctly describe the body as a system that adjusts constantly to its environment by means of complex feedback mechanisms. These minor fluctuations in body states, such as increase of healthy adaptive processes. From the physiological point of view, death is always the result of disease. The organism seems to have been made to exist forever, always recovering from any malfunction through its ingenious system of adaptation. The organism dies as a result of injuries inflicted upon it by the environment, and not from any intrinsic cause.

The ontological concept of disease perceives death somewhat differently. From this point of view, an organism may have homeostatic properties, but its powers of self-maintenance have their limits. Consequently, when the environment stresses, the organism pasts its ability to cope with such stress, the organism is unable to survive. Ontologically speaking, disease can be viewed as discrete entities, such as plaque, pollution or radiation sickness. Without disease and death, natural evolution cannot continue.

Two other theories regarding disease have had considerable impact on current medical thought. These are the mechanistic and the organismic theories of disease.

The mechanistic theory has influenced many modern medical educators and biologists. For these workers, the parts of an organism are perceived as being more significant and controllable than the whole. Their work has been that of isolating the physical and anatomical hallmarks of disease and studying trends among specific disease forms. For instance, gastroenterologists will study the characteristics of such diseases as acute cholecystitis or gastric ulcers diseases affecting the gall bladder and the stomach, respectively. Their approach to a patient with the stomach ache will involve isolating and identifying the patient's disease. Having identified the patient's problem as, say, acute cholecystisis, they go about treating it according to the rules they have set for the treatment of acute cholecystisis.

In effect, practitioners whose perception of disease is mechanistic run the risk of concentrating too much on treating the problem and not the patient. This risk would seem to be particularly significant for those in the medical specialties and subspecialties. Medical specialization should be accompanied by comprehensive holistic medical knowledge.

Other healthcare workers view disease in terms of relationship between the parts that make up the human being. This is the organismic theory of disease, which emphasizes that the relationship among the parts of the body are just as real and scientifically observable as the anatomy of the parts themselves. It also stresses that in understanding disease, the parts of the body cannot be understood in isolation but in the context of the system in which they exist. One healing tradition which takes an organismic approach to disease and concentrates on reestablishing the harmonious relationship between vital body forces in Chinese Traditional Medicine.

CHAPTER
3

TREASURE HERBS-MIRACLES FROM CHANGBAI MOUNTAIN-A PLACE WHERE THE EXCELLENT NATURAL CHINESE MEDICINE EVOLVED

THE IDEA OF USING CHINESE MEDICINE TO CURE THE MOST SERIOUS DISEASE CANCER

DEEPEST REGRET AFTER SEEING A TERMINAL CANCER PATIENT

"DOCTOR, please help my mom! please!"

A girl crying rushed to me and kneeled in from of me as I was passing by the ward. I stood beside the bed looking at the dying mother and the crying daughter and I could not do anything.

I had just graduated from the medical school (Tonghua City School of Sanitation, Jilin Province) and I was an intern (Liudaokuo College of Sanitation). As I passed through the cancer ward, a girl stopped me for she mistook me for a doctor because of my white uniform.

Her mother was in her early forties and was hospitalized because of terminal liver cancer. Her abdomen was swollen as if she was pregnant and she had no more than two weeks to live.

The Chief doctor had already told her to accept the fact that her mother is dying The daughter who could never accept the loss of her suffering mother was staring at her. As natural reaction, she screamed for help as she saw me.

I thought it was too late to help her mother and she died a week later in October of 1972.

Although I was only an intern, I felt helpless as I saw the daughter making every effort to save her mother. Instead of wiping tears from her face, I just cried with her.

What is cancer? I thought I know a little now. But then I knew it was an incurable disease and patients who were admitted to the hospital after having been diagnosed of cancer were facing death.

However, when I witnessed the death of the mother, I pondered "Is cancer really incurable?"

I doubted it. It was on that day of my youth that I decided 'I would never let this happen again, I must cure cancer."

I vowed inside my heart.

It was my long life desire to cure cancer some twenty-six years ago. It was early autumn of my nineteenth year.

Treasure of herbs- an honor to be in Changbai Mountain

I was born in a remote mountain village near Tonghua in Northeastern China (Manchuria) not far from the border between Jilin Province and North Korea.

I will tell you the story about the place where I was born and the experiences of my youth. They are the inspiration for my becoming a doctor and were the bases for my belief that cancer can be cured with Chinese medicine. In other words, it is the start of a quest and not the story of my achievements.

It takes a whole day and night to travel from Beijing to Tonghua City by train. It is a remote city in Northeastern part of China. It is well known because there are many Japanese immigrants in the area and most of them settled in the capital, Changchun, Tonghua which is the third largest city in the province of Jilin.

Tonghua lies almost on the same latitude of Hakodate, Japan. Situated in the Changbai Mountains, it snows during winter and the temperature sometimes can fall to 30 degrees below zero.

The central mountain of the Changbai Mountain range is also called the street of Chinese medicine. People including the Japanese were always coming to buy Chinese medicine. It explains why Changbai Mountain has long been referred to as the "treasure of herbs" and considered the homeland of Chinese medicine.

Detailed description about Changbai Mountain and its herbs are presented in later chapters. The mountain has been a volcano since ancient times. In winter, the whole area is covered with snow and the natural habitat is preserved fertile environment for making herbs.

I was born in Gungyi Village, a rural city of Tonghua surrounded by Changbai Mountains. I am the second son among six children. We were poor and all eight members of the family lived in a small humble two-room house whose income is derived from farming.

During that time, we began working in the fields when we were six or seven years old. No matter how hard we worked, the whole village was still poor and we could only get a meager income.

Although life was difficult, we were lucky to be surrounded by the Changbai Mountains for they are the few places in China where precious herbs can be found. As a child, I learned from the adults how to gather herbs.

In just a short time, I could identify over a hundred kind of herbs!

Then I learned how to identify these valuable herbs and I began serious efforts to save them. After a half-day's work, I would go to Tonghua City to sell them.

My father was elated. I did not only help support the family but also saved enough to pay for my tuition in the junior high school. After two to three years, I was very confused. I could make only a small fortune by gathering herbs. The village remained poor and we had no doctors. It was not an easy task to gather herbs and people were forced to sell them in order to feed their families.

It was during those years of confusion that I graduated from the junior high school. During that time, my mother suffered severe abdominal pain. I believed it was acute gastritis and I gave her a prescription according to my knowledge and experience in herbs identification. In just a few days, my mother recovered and returned to the field to work.

"The herb really cures!"

I told myself, "I need to save lives and cure illnesses... I want to be a doctor!"

It was the dream of an innocent youth.

REALIZATION OF A DREAM 'TO BE A DOCTOR'

Reality is cruel! To be a doctor became elusive for people who come from a poor village. No one would dare to say it.

After I graduated from high school, my big brother inherited my father's property. I went to work on a pig farm but I still continued collecting herbs during my spare time. Collecting herbs became more difficult because I don't trade with them in order to begin my research.

I did not want to grow pigs for the rest of my life. I wanted to learn more about herbs and I needed to be a doctor. I wanted to realize my dream.

I used half of my first wages to buy an illustrated book of herbs, "The Herbs in Northeastern China." It was worth it as it broadened the horizons of my life. This book is still on the shelf.

The book contains detailed descriptions about the variety, combination, functions and effects of the herbs.

Then I documented the herbs as directed in the book, and I put them in bottles according to their categories.

I asked myself, "Are my prescriptions as effective as stated in the book? Can they cure human diseases?" The more I think, the more I want to try.

At that time, I learned that an elder in the village was suffering from bronchial asthma and I went directly to his place. I already had a prescription for the ailment.

Because he knew and trusted me, he agreed to use the medicine to do me a favor. It worked for 3 days and a month later, he returned to the field to work.

Diarrhea was common in the village. After using my prescriptions, people were cured.

I have earned people's recognition because of my knowledge of herbs and their healing powers.

At the pig's farm, I was promoted assistant veterinary. I began to learn more Chinese medicine practices. The first was acupuncture.

I became an esteemed member of the village after my prescriptions have been discovered effective.

The people began spreading the word. "There is a young man in Gungyi Village who is an expert in acupuncture and herbal medicine and he has cured the diseases of many villagers."

Through word of mouth from the villagers, the message fell upon the ears of Director Wang, Ming-Te of the People's Commune Sanitation College, and he invited me to study there. It was a big opportunity.

I started my lifelong career. The College provided me with training in Chinese and Western Medicines.

I wanted very much to study in Beijing but coming from a poor family the dream seemed impossible. After six months at the College, I got a lucky break.

The People's Government planned to build special medical schools in remote areas and it gave birth to Tonghua School of Sanitation, the place where I was born.

After graduation, I was required to stay there for a year. It gave me a chance to study both Chinese and Western medicines systematically.

I became an intern at the Liudoukuo hospital where I met the crying girl and the dying mother.

It was at that point that I made up my mind I must use my beloved herbs to cure cancer!

Had I known more about cancer, its enigma, its complexities, and its ubiquitousness, I would have been more informed.

I thought, "I will win the Nobel Prize when I invent a new panacea for cancer." An award still elusive to many cancer researchers. Being young, courageous, passionate and fearless, I was consumed with the desire to conquer cancer.

TO CURE CANCER WITH TRADITONAL CHINESE HERBS

Youth and passion are two most beautiful privileges one can have. When I decided to challenge cancer, I was still an intern. The death of the crying girl's mother served as the inspiration.

42

I have always thought that cancer can be cured by using Chinese Medicine natural remedy.

Then I tried to combine Chinese medicine with herbal medicine from Japan.

Chinese medicine is of course indispensable in the area where I was born.

None of these treatments have any relation with scientific or medical advancements. Cancer treatment by Western medicine could not be everything. Even with all the researches and advanced technologies, a cure for fatal cancer has not yet been found.

Both doctors and scholars agree that no definitive treatment for cancer exists. For instance, surgical operations, radiation treatments, and chemotherapy have many harmful side effects and cannot prevent the spread from one organ to another. There is no cure for terminal cancer.

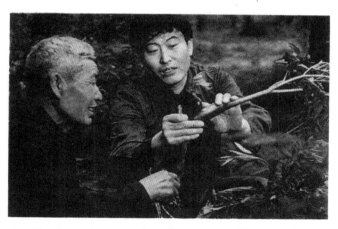

Dr. Wang looked for good herbs and prescription in China when he was young.

CLASSIFYING 1200 KINDS OF HERBS AND PRESCRIPTIONS WITH CHINESE MEDICINE THEORIES

I classified my collection according to Chinese medicine theories including their advantages and disadvantages as well as their characteristics.

The terms, 'raw medicine', 'herbs', and 'Chinese medicines' in this book have different definitions. Here is a description.

'Raw medicine' refers to plants, animals and minerals used for medical purposes. It becomes a medicine after drying and simple processing.

Herbs refer to plants. Chinese medicine sometimes refers to single raw medicine or combined medications to form prescriptions. Therefore, most raw medicines and Chinese medicines are herbs.

Unless otherwise stated, both raw medicine and Chinese medicine are synonymous.

After classification and documentation, I began studying each prescription according to its real effects and functions. In other words, after confirming the advantages and disadvantages of each kind of raw medicine, I tried to find out whether raw medicines and prescriptions were effective in higher dosages or with prolonged use.

I used the Chinese medicine theories as my framework of classification. It is believed that the body is composed of three elements-space energy, blood and water.

In simple terms, energy refers to the very thing that sustains one's life. Blood is the source of nutrition and water is present in the human body. It is called lymph liquid in Western medicine.

In Chinese medicine, when the body's overall flow slows down, diseases can take hold and a human body will become dry and a disease will be formed. Therefore, maintaining a smooth flow of energy, blood and

Different prescriptions have different effects. Doctors are referred as geniuses if they are able to invent different workable prescriptions according to signs and symptoms. Therefore, in Chinese medicine, a pharmacist is more important than a physician and the best description should come from pharmacists' ingenuity.

Raw medicine is incredible! For instance, we can prescribe two raw medicines of diverse functions at an equal of different proportion, or we can add other raw medicines in the prescription. By doing this we can dramatically increase the effects. In other words, if the effect of a single raw medicine is striking, the combination of two or more medicines will greatly enhance the effect.

The common *Radix Puerariae Soup* used for the common cold is prescribed chiefly with the root of *Pueraria, Lobata* together with *ephedra, ginger, red date, cinnamon peel, paeonia albiflora var hortensis, and liquorice.*

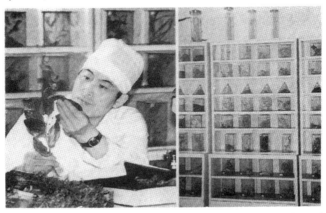

We carefully chose some 30 raw medicines from over 60 selection for further evaluation.

Radix Puerariae Soup is still a common prescription in Chinese medicine. I have learned the secrets of over 2,000 years of Chinese medicine in accordance with the four basic principles. The *"Typhoid Theory,* which records the use of over 100 kinds of raw medicines was written by *Zhang Zhong Jiing,* the father of Chinese medicine. It contains complete history and description of Chinese medicine.

First, I chose 60 raw medicines containing anti cancer properties from the original 1,200 samples. In accordance with the four principles, I continued to study them. After I concluded a series of tests on guinea pigs, I selected 30 from the chosen 60 subjects.

Then I spent two more years experimenting and testing different variations on the final 30 subjects. After countless trial and error, I finally developed my anti cancer Chinese medicine.

Most of the final 30 subjects produce high anti cancer effects. They help strengthen the gastrointestinal system, facilitate urination, promote body condition and improve immunity. The functions of each of the final 30 subjects have been clearly recorded.

To avert metastasis of cancer and to demonstrate synergy and multiple effects of the medicine, over a thousand clinical trials have been done before the final prescription came out.

However, the prototype was as big as a duck's egg. After reformulating the contents and dosage, I finally developed the capsule. After the success of the 110-capsule, I still kept on improving it and thus developed the new China No. 1 Tian Xian Liquid.

It is named after the two major raw medicines used in the liquid, the *Radix Trichosnthis and Radix Clematidis.*

CLINICAL EXPERIMENTS AT TIANJIN PHARMACOLOGY INSTITUTE PROVE POSITIVE EFFECTS

Continuous experiments and tests were conducted on guinea pigs and tests were applied on tumors were performed to improve the product until we were sure that it was effective against cancer.

Then we began to perform human tests of the China No.1 Tian Xian Capsule in rural hospitals. However, most hospitals believed in Western medicine. Some doctors questioned the efficacy of Chinese medicine to cure cancer. But some doctors have been trained in Chinese medicine so I begged them to try China No.1 Tian Xian Capsule. No official reply was received at that time. It is categorized as a kind of secret prescription and doctors would not accept it because of pride and prejudice. Failure was a natural consequence.

As a person who never surrender, I began looking for cancer patients diagnosed by hospitals to recommend the capsule to them.

However, can a stranger convince a cancer patient to use the capsule? At this point, it was only I who was devoted to the research. I had made no contacts with mainstream medicine. From these few facts, I realized the cruel reality caused by my lack of knowledge and recognition from the authority of big hospitals.

In the greatest moment of my despair, an old man from my hometown with his family came to me upon hearing that I was looking for subjects to try my new medicine. He said to me, "I am suffering from terminal stomach cancer, even doctors have given me up. I am so frustrated and hopeless . I heard that you give medicine for free, can I try? I won't blame you even if I die."

I felt sorry for him. I was very excited to have a willing subject. I held his hands and gave him a bottle of China No.1 Tian Xian Capsule.

A month later, his family came very happy and informed me that the pain has disappeared and he is getting better and stronger. Two months later, the old man sent me a letter together with his latest diagnosis. It showed that the tumor had disappeared, regained his appetite and he could even perambulate.

It was very touching that my body was shaken up not because of the proof of the letter but because of a 'miracle'. I will never forget that day, I was 29 years old. It has been 11 years since I devoted myself to research on July 12, 1984.

The old man who had miraculous remission with China No.1 Tian Xian Capsule spread it by word of mouth and those who needed help came incessantly. Some were cured, some were not, however, most users said that all cancer patients were alleviated in some ways which means that some terminal cancer patients died peacefully. Families of many patients have traveled great distances to express their gratitude to me.

Then I consolidated all clinical reports and sent them to large hospitals in Beijing and none of them showed interest. I knew it was due to lack of expert's approval who in authority.

It was at that time general secretary of the Tonghua City Office became a witness to the efficacy of China No. 1 Tian Xian Capsule who tried to arrange clinical experiments and tests with credible hospitals especially the Tianjin Pharmacology Research Institution.

Six months later, a reply from the institution came confirming the true effects of the China No. 1 Tian Xian Capsule.

To tell the truth, I was very confident because my research showed nearly two-thirds of the 50 subjects claimed that the capsule was effective.

I had also confidence in the raw medicines used in the capsule. They are shown in Table 1. It shows the contents of each capsule.

All raw medicines used in the capsule were gathered from my hometown. They are all herbs from Changbai Mountain. The miraculous effect of the anti cancer herbs from the 'treasure of herbs' unbelievable!

Table 1: Major Contents and Properties of China No. 1 Tian Xian Capsule

Raw	Medicine Functions
Radix Trichosanthis	[Material] roots of Trichosanthis and Kirilowii Maxim [function] anti-tumor, anti-bacterial
Radix Clematidis	[material] roots of clematis of Chinensis Osbeck [function] pain-reliever, anti-bacterial, anti-tumor.
Black Nightshade	[material] Black Nightshade of the eggplant [function] anti-tumor, anti-inflammation, anti-bacteria, improves heart functions and blood pressure
Seu Hedysari	[material] root of Radix Astragali Seu Hedysari of beans [function] reduces blood pressure, improves immunity, anti-bacteria, facilitate urination
Ginseng	[material] root of ginseng of Panax Ginseng C.A. Mey. [function] strengthens stomach, supplements energy, and improve body functions.
Polyprous Umbellata	[material] Polyprous Umbellata fungi of spongiform fungi. [function] improves immunity, anti-tumor, facilitate uri nation, kills germs.
Venenum Bufonis	[material] toad Venenum Bufonis. [function] removes poisonous substances, relieves pain.
Calsulus Bovis	[material] gall and gall stone of cow. [function] strengthens heart, relieves pain, removes body heat, remove poisonous substances.

TREASURE OF HERBS - MIRACLES FROM CHANGBAI MOUNTAIN BRING EXCELLENT CHINESE MEDICINE

Changbai Mountain is an active volcano which lies on the Chinese-Korean border located in the middle of Tunghua River Douman River and Yalu River, with an elevation of 2744m. Koreans call it the *White Head Mountain* , and Japanese named it Changbai Mountain (according to the Japanese dictionary Kouzien).

I have mentioned many times in this book that Changbai Mountain has long been referred to as the 'treasure of herbs' and the 'hometown of Chinese medicine'. In other words, I was not only born in the best place but also with the best environment for Chinese medicine research. I cannot help but be proud of my country. Here is a brief description of the medicines in Changbai Mountain.

There are over 6,000 kinds of natural herbs in China, and they are too many to study. It is known that there are over 1300 kinds growing in Changbai Mountain.

Nowadays, herbs of Changbai Mountain are under government control and gathering is prohibited. Therefore, excellent herbs can be preserved.

Why do I keep emphasizing that herbs from Changbai Mountain are the best? It is because of the soil and ecology of the mountain. It is located near the crater and the ashes from the eruptions produced fertile soils.

For centuries, the soil has absorbed the nutrition and minerals of the ashes to form fertile contents of the soil. For example, selenium and germanium are two very important micro elements to human body and they are found here in high levels. They are elements used to ameliorate the body's condition.

In addition, the snows on the mountain act as freezing agents in preserving the soil. Winter is longer than summer so that plants have longer time to 'sleep' and it is an essential factor in producing excellent herbs. As herbs are considered plants, they are subjected to different environmental growing conditions. The nutrition, quality, and quantity of effective substances inside the plants are always different. The water and nutrition from the roots, the photosynthesis, the soil, and temperature all affect the plants.

According to the research report of Dr. Hamilton in the United Kingdom, he asserts that herbs grown in tough environment and harsh climate will contain 2 to 3 times more potencies than herbs grown in warmer areas.

The same theory can be applied to anti-cancer contents, the same herbs from Changbai Mountain will have different qualities than those grown in other places.

For instance, the anti-cancer content in herb called *mandragonrine* from Changbai Mountain is 2.5 times greater than samples from Hebei.

This is not a new fact about Changbai Mountain. There is a volcanic lake on the mountain called *Tian Chyr* and the water contains high levels of micro elements.

Here is an example. To produce Korean ginseng wine, people get water from Tian Chyr and after they put the dried ginseng inside, the wine become distilled. They discovered that the dried ginseng begins to sprout, an effect not observed when placed in ordinary rice wine. It shows that waters from Tian Chyr contain element that enlivens the plants.

However, it is nothing special to the local folks.

In fact, the waters of Changbai Mountain used for Korean ginseng are daily necessities of the local folks who tend to have lived very long lives. The 'longlife village' is famous far and wide and the fact that many of the people are over 80 to 100 years old are not due to miracles. The water and soil of Changbai Mountain make the place more mysterious and continue to stir the people's imagination.

I am very proud to have completed the major task of my mission in my hometown in Changbai Mountain. I just want you to know that without the herbs of Changbai Mountain neither China No.1 Tian Xian Capsule nor China No.1 Tian Xian Liquid would be a success.

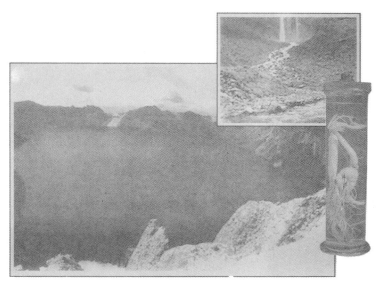

Treasure of herbs'-Changbai Mountain, water from the volcano lake Tian Chyr can make dried ginseng sprout.

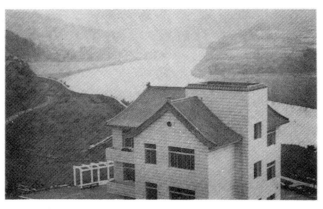

Tonghua Changbai Mountain Pharmacology Research Institution, Center of Research of the herbs from the mountain.

CHAPTER

4

POWER IN AUTHORITY APPROVES AND GOVERNMENT APPROVES ANTI CANCER NATURAL CHINESE MEDICINE

PRC NATIONAL RESEARCH PROJECT SELECTED, GOVERNMENT-APPROVED ANTI CANCER MEDICATION

LARGE SCALE CLINICAL TEST PROCEEDED AS NATIONAL RESEARCH PROJECT

AFTER ELEVEN years, my dreams gradually materialized after I decided to use traditional Chinese medicine to cure cancer.

The first recognition of my China No.1 Tian Xian Capsule as an effective anti cancer medication came from the National Tianjin Pharmacology Research Institution. At present, I keep on improving China No. 1 Tian Xian Liquid. Details will be given in later sections. The milestones in research and development of China No. 1 Tian Xian Liquid are listed below.

1983	Completion of China No. 1 Tian Xian Capsule.
1984	Published Clinical test of the Tianjin Pharmacology Research Institution.
1986	Selected as an item of the National Scientific and Technological Development Program. Official research

project began.

1986   Established and directed the Tonghua Changbai Mountain Anti Cancer Medicine Research Institute.

1987   Established the Jilin Province Anti cancer Association and the Changbai Mountain.

1988   80% effective curative rate approved by clinical tests done by the US Cancer Center

1988   China No. 1 Tian Xian Capsule first approved by the Chinese Government as an effective anti cancer medication.

1991   Completion of China No. 1 Tian Xian Liquid.

1995   Improvement of China No. 1 Tian Xian Liquid completed.

1997   Further researches fortified China No. 1 Tian Xian Liquid.

After approval by the Tianjin Pharmacology Research Institution, the general use of China No. 1 Tian Xian Liquid for cancer patients started. As the number of users increased, the effectiveness of the China No. 1 Tian Xian Capsule spread and attracted the attention of hospitals and medical institutions.

In 1985, Profs. Lee Der Hwa and Yu Guey Ching formed a research team to conduct another clinical test and experiment of China No. 1 Tian Xian Capsule. The result pointed out that the capsule had considerable effect on cancer patient, and was more reputed than in previous reports.

Test here refers to the survey on the nature and capacity of a subject, experiment on the examination of the theory under certain conditions. To avoid unnecessary troubles, the term 'clinical test' will be used for the rest of the chapter in the book unless otherwise stated.

After the assessment, Tianjin Pharmacology Research Institution gave it a 'valuable national research'. The government has accepted China No. 1 Tian Xian Capsule as an item of the Government's Scientific and Technological Development Program. In other words, the capsule was developed as a new anti cancer medication which was already a national research project.

The first program started three years ago after the completion of the capsule in 1986.

After the experiments at the Tianjin Pharmacology Research Institution, clinical tests then proceeded on to China's Chinese Medicine Research Institute at Guagan Hospital followed by twenty five other medical institutions and schools all over China.

The program has three goals : clinical test on cancer patients after using the capsule, pharmacological tests of the capsule; and mass production of the new anti cancer medication. During the program, I was chosen to be the chief researcher of the government-founded Tonghua Changbai Mountain Anti Cancer Medication Research Institute.

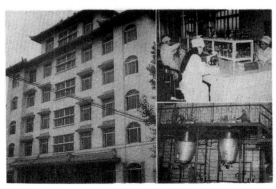

Facilities at Jilin Anticancer Association, Changbai Mountain Pharmacology Research institute, include a factory

In 1987, China No. 1 Tian Xian Capsule received high acclaim for its efficacy. After developing ways of mass production, the government has deemed it wise to make the original research institute my personal research institute. Maybe it was a result of waves of reform. The Institute changed its name to Jilin Anti Cancer Association, Changbai Mountain Pharcology Institute.

THE FIRST GOVERNMENT-RECOGNIZED ANTI CANCER MEDICATION

Not long after being Chair of the Jilin Anti Cancer Association Changbai Mountain Pharmacology Institute, the project team determined the aforementioned three goals a remarkable accomplishment. Recognition from the society came incessantly. Then I applied a license for the anti-cancer capsule to the Public Health Department. However, it was at that time when the government was amending health and medical policies, the government would not issue a license for medication without presenting an inspection certification and accreditation.

Therefore, the team initiated a new clinical test to secure a license for a new anti cancer medication. About a year later, 287 out of the total of 511 subjects using the capsule showed there was no need for operation, radiation therapy or chemotherapy. In other words, the reduction or disappearance of the tumors were confirmed. Other tests on the capsule was conducted such as the combined use of radiotherapy and/or chemotherapy while pharmacological and toxic tests were also performed at the same time.

According to the aforementioned clinical tests, we obtained data about the capsule; as effective anti cancer medication, pain reliever, immunity improvement, extension of life; no side effect on blood functions, heart, liver, kidney. We immediately applied for a new license.

In September of 1988, the official name of China No. 1 Tian Xian Capsule came out and the license as an anti cancer medication was granted by the government. The Jilin Tonghua Changbai Mountain Pharmaceutical Factory began the official production and the product was distributed to appointed cancer clinics.

Through continuous research and development, we began to make a liquid form. This is the present Improved China No. 1 Tian Xian Liquid.

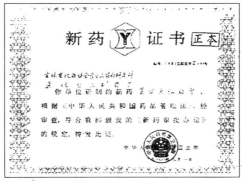

The medicine of Anti-Cancer, recognized by the Ministry of Public Health of China

MANY MEDICAL INSTITUTIONS HAVE OBTAINED TREATMENT RATE OF 80%

Three years after having been chosen as national research project, continuous clinical tests proceeded in 25 medical institutions and schools throughout China.

Those tests had provided us with all kinds of data. Since the data was too complex and technical, only one example is given here in terms of illustration. For example, esophagus and stomach cancer patients were using the capsule for 4-6 consecutive months. (Please refer to Table 2)

The figure shows that 80.2% condition of the esophagus and stomach of cancer patients has changed after receiving China No. 1 Tian Xian capsule.

Mild refers to the disappearance of the tumor, better referred as reduction or partial disappearance of the tumor, and stable refers to stoppage of cancer cell multiplication. The total rate of the three items is referred to as the effective rate.

The result of the clinical tests is: mild 1.2%; better 2.0%; and stable 77.0%, the total is 80.2%.

The most important point is that 77.0% of the patients became stable. It means the tumor has been reduced and no metastasis occured. If no further treatment is given, cancer cells will once again multiply. When there is no sign of multiplication, it means possibility of cure. Many medical institutions commented that "it's wonderful to have an efficacy rate at 80%." It is the most credible comment about the capsule.

Table 2: Treatment Results of China No. 1 Tian Xian Capsule on Esophagus and Stomach Cancer Patients

	Subjects	Mild	Better	Stable	Progress
Esophagus Cancer	172	2	5	129	36
		1.2%	2.9%	75.0%	20.9%
Stomach Cancer	177	2	2	140	33
		1.15%	1.15%	79.1%	18.6%
Total	349	4	7	269	69
		1.2%	2.0%	77.0%	19.8%

Mild: tumor disappears or reduces by over 50%

Better: tumor reduces by 25%-50%

Stable: tumor reduces less than 25% (no new tumor is located)

GOOD RESULTS FROM THE CLINICAL TESTS COMPLETED AT THE U.S. CANCER CENTER

Upon progression of the national scale clinical tests, Prof. Lee Deer Hwa introduced me to two researchers at the International Cancer Convention in Beijing.

At that time, the anti cancer effect of the China No. 1 Tian Xian Capsule had become a hot subject in the Chinese medical circle and among patients. It also attracted the attention of scholars from Japan, USA and Canada. Two scholars have given their highest respect to the research. One was an overseas Chinese, Dr. Lee Yuh Chwan from RTI Institute, North Carolina and another one was Dr. Robert Schmitt from the US Cancer Center.

'We want to make further research on China No. 1 Tian Xian Capsule, may we read all the related data?'

I handed out all the data, and after the clinical tests have been done by the US Cancer Center, the capsule was proven to be effective.

I learned of the result two years later in 1988. I was giving a speech on the effects of the capsule among terminal cancer patients in Japan. An invitation from the US Cancer Center urged me to continue my speech on the anti cancer effects of Radix Trichosanthis and Radix Clematidis in USA.

It was after the speech that Dr. Schmitt had informed me of the result. The tests were done on guinea pigs with 48 kinds of cancer cells.

According to Dr. Schmitt, the capsule had an effective rate at 80.4% on 48 kinds of cancer cells. It shows that the result from the US Cancer Center is almost the same as that China. The result from the US Cancer Center did relieve me, despite my confidence.

Since it is official, here are some important points of the result.

1. Free of acute toxins
2. Effective in increasing the white blood cells and immunity of white blood cell
3. Effective in increasing the hemoglobin
4. Improves immunity
5. High suppression effect on S 180j cancer cell
6. Effective rate at 48.1% on intestinal cancer
7. High prevention to cancer cells on guinea pigs
8. 64% spread control on lung cancer
9. Suppresses expanding liver cancer
10. Considerate effect when combined with radiotherapy

The results of the effectiveness and principles of the new anti cancer medication are the raw medicines used in the capsule which can effectively control the growth of cancer cells, block composition of the protein necessary for cancer cell growth, suppress the DNA composition of cancer cells, etc. They strengthen the immunity of white blood cells.

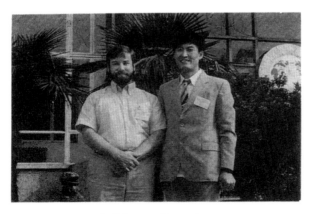

Dr. Schmitt and the author

Improving and Strengthening China No. 1 Tian Xian Capsule and China No. 1 Tian Xian Liquid

The clinical tests and pharmacological study validated that the project was a success so that we moved on to mass production of the product and started making it into liquid.

Prof. Wang Zhen-Guo was awarded the Supreme Honor for the Best Individual Invention during the 38th Eureka Invention Expo held in Brussells, Belguim.

Everyone knows that the liquid is easier absorbed in the stomach than the pill. Therefore, converting the capsule into liquid is very important.

The clinical tests of the capsule posed some problems; one is the difficulty in using the capsule to treat some cancers.

For instance, it is difficult for terminal cancer patients to ingest capsule. The capsule irritates the throat due to quantity of dosage.

Moreover, it takes longer time for a capsule to dissolve then for it will cause acidity, nausea, vomiting, and even diarrhea.

Liquid then is the best solution. After reviewing the results of the clinical tests and the pharmacological study, we opted to formulate a better dosage with different ingredients.

For instance, in order to liquify the capsule, we developed a new idea for quality ingredients, new formula, etc. Basically, the ingredients are the same as that of the capsule, but we wanted a better medicine.

Regarding quality of the ingredients, I must emphasize that all raw medicines must come from Changbai Mountain.

It is a proven fact that extracts from fresh herbs are more effective than those from dried herbs. It is the same in animal raw medicine.

Therefore, the Changbai Mountain Pharmacology Research Institute decided only to use fresh herbal and animal extracts to develop the medicine.

It took three years to improve and modify the China No. 1 Tian Xian Capsule into liquid form. It is the first liquid anti cancer Chinese medicine so I named it China No. 1 Tian Xian Liquid. When it is combined with China No. 1 Tian Xian Capsule, the effects accelerate but the liquid form is much easier to take.

China No. 1 Tian Xian Liquid was immediately sent to hospitals and medical schools in Beijing, Tianjin and Jilin for clinical tests. Table 3 shows higher than expected efficacy rates found from 699 subjects suffering from seven kinds of cancer.

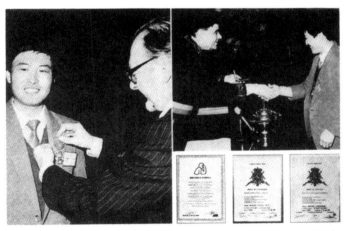

Awarded the World's Best Individual Invention Price in the 38th Eureke World in Invention Expo.

Table 3: Effects of Treatment of China No. 1 Tian Xian Liquid on Terminal Cancers

Cancer	Patients	Success	Failure
Esophagus	225	201	24
Stomach	376	334	42
Intestine	95	85	10
Subtotal	696	620	76
Lung	94	73	21
Liver	34	25	9
Breast	78	56	22
Brain	46	28	18

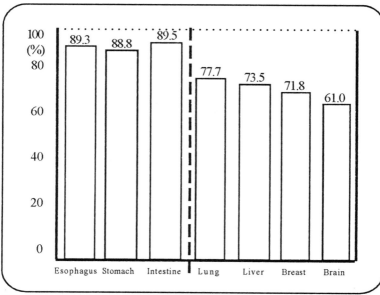

The effective rate on the firs three was a high as 90%

The clinical tests show that China No. 1 Tian Xian Liquid is more effective than China No.1 Tian Xian Capsule.

Both the liquid and capsule forms of China No.1 Tian Xian series received the Best Product Award in the Asia Pacific Region, the Golden Award from the 2nd Beijing International Product Exposition, and the Best Personal Achievement Award in the 38th Eureka Invention Expo.

Upon completion of China No. 1 Tian Xian Liquid, Chancellor JIANG-min visited the remote Jilin Anti Cancer Association, Changbai Mountain Pharmacology Research Institute in Tonghua to recognize my achievement.

It has been 15 years since the development of the China No. 1 Tian Xian Capsule, and constant developments have resulted in the Improved China No. 1 Tian Xian Liquid. It all started from 1200 herbs narrowing to 60, then to 30, and down to the final 20, which are used in our 'miracle prescriptions.' The major ingredients and their functions (the latest generation China No. 1 Tian Xian Liquid) are listed in Table 4. We hope readers will understand that it is a product of many different raw medicines containing various properties.

One must bear in mind that this is not a complete list of raw ingredients, a few were omitted as they are our 'commercial secrets.' Since the introduction of the prototype in 1991, everything has been approved by the government in the following years.

This has nothing to do with secrecy. Had we disclosed all the formula at a time the dysfunctional legal system has laxed policies it would have resulted in countless counterfeits. In order to prevent any harm to the reputation of the product, I only revealed the formula to trustworthy government departments. Of course, the formula is public knowledge as imitation of the same product is impossible although, counterfeits and homogeneous products are unavoidable. As I have mentioned before, all ingredients used in the product are raw medicines from Changbai Mountain including the animal medicines. The animals used are raised inside my Institute in Tonghua.

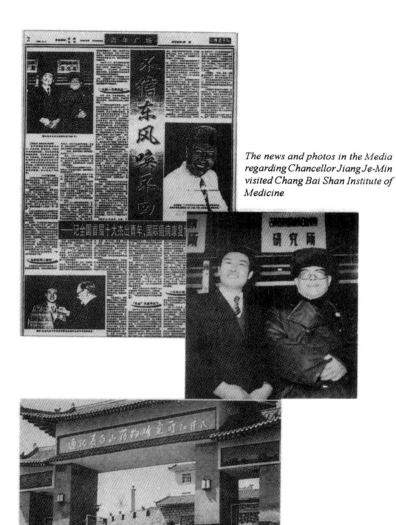

The news and photos in the Media regarding Chancellor Jiang Je-Min visited Chang Bai Shan Institute of Medicine

CHANCELLOR JIANG wrote the banner above the entrance of the Changbai Mountain Pharmacology Research Institute. The completion of the research enabled us to celebrate the accomplishment of the national project.

73

IT IS 'SIDE-EFFECT' FREE ANTI CANCER CHINESE MEDICINE

At present, the most common cancer treatments in Western medicine are surgical operations, radiation therapy and chemotherapy. However, none of them have positive effects. During operations, the affected area is removed to prevent the spread of cancer to other areas but to no avail. The only solution is to remove a large part of an organ, including unaffected tissues. In doing so, the original functions of the organs have been greatly affected.

Radiation therapy and chemotherapy kill as many healthy cells as cancer cells in the process. Therefore, they cause dramatic side effects. This is the handicap of Western medicine.

The combined use of the radiotherapy and chemotherapy with China No. 1 Tian Xian Liquid is described in Chapter IV, and here is a brief introduction to the side effects.

According to statistics, normal, healthy and fast-growing cells are killed in a radiotherapy and chemotherapy. For example, the tissues of digestive organs, blood cells, and capillaries of marrow are all affected.

The side effects include uneasiness, vomiting, diarrhea, bloody stool, oral cavity ulcers, anemia, agranulocytosis, and hair loss. On top of the common cancer symptoms, there is difficulty in swallowing, loss of appetite and loss of weight. A cancer patient suffers not only physical pain but also mental distress during treatments. Normally, the side effects damage the normal cells which is turn affects the immune system and subsequently reduce the body's natural resistance to infection. Therefore, common colds can easily result to pneumonia, viral infections and profuse bleeding.

Table 4: Major Raw Medicines and Effects of China No. 1 Tian Xian Liquid

Ingredients	Material and Effect
Ginseng	[Material]: root of Panax Ginseng C.A. Mey [Effect]: improves all body functions.
Pearl	[Material]: shell pearl [Effect]: anti-allergy, keeps concentration, facilitates metabolism
Astrayali seu Hedysari	[Material]: root of Radix Astrayali Seu Hedysari [Effect]: extends blood vessels, lowers blood pressure, improves immunity, anti-bacteria, facilitates urination, removes excretion
Black Nightshade	[Material]: leaves of Black Nightshade, a kind of eggplant. [Effect]: anti cancer, anti-inflammation, anti-bacteria, strengthens heart, lowers blood pressure
.Borneolum	[Material]: resin of Borneolum Syntheticum plants [Effect]: relieves pain, anti-inflammation, improves blood circulation.
Syntheticum	[Material]: root and bundle of Syntheticum [Effect]: lowers blood sugar, anti-bacteria, anti-bruise, anti-lumps, facilitates urination, suppresses sweating.
Trichosanthis	[Material]: root of Trichosnathis and Kirilowii Maxim. [Effect]: anti-tumor, anti bacteria
Radix Clemantidis	[Material]: root of Clemantis of Chinensis Osbeck [Effect]: relieves pain, anti-bacteria, anti cancer of digestive organs
Herba Hedjotis Diffusae	[Material]: root of Herba Hedyotis Diffusae [Effect]: improves immunity, anti cancer, improves suprarenal gland functions.
Indigo Naturalis	[Material]: dry color of Baphicacunthus cusia Bremek [Effect]: anti-tumor, protects liver, improves digestive function, anti-bacteria.
Fructus Ligustri Lucidi	[Material]: fruit of Ligustrum Lucidum Ait. [Effect] : reduces fat in blood vessels, strengthens heart, facilitates urination, suppresses cough, im proves immunity, anti bacteria.

Liquorice	[Material]: root and bundle of liquorice of bean
	[Effect]: controls immunity, relieves pain, suppresses cough, anti digestive ulcer, anti-inflammation
Polyporus	[Material]: dried fungi nuclei of Polyporus Umbellata, a kind of spongi form fungus
Umbellata	[Effect]: Polyporus Umbellata extract and Polyporus Umbellata polysaccharide improves immunity, anti tumor, facilitates urination and anti bacteria
Animal Gall Juice	[Material]: animal gall bladder
	[Effect]: relieves pain, anti parasites.
Animal Excretion	[Material]: dried excretion of male animals
	[Effect]: anti-bacteria, improves heart blood flow, excites heart muscle, anti tumor, relieves pain.

Table 5: Toxin Reaction Test on China No. 1 Tian Xian Capsule

	0	1	II	III IV	
Subject (349)	232	105	12	0	1
%	66.5%	30.1%	3.4%	0%	0%

Remarks: Toxin Reaction Distinction

O: not toxin reaction is found

I: slight toxin reaction, within the tolerance of patients, no need to stop using medication.

II: detectable toxin reaction affecting organ functions, medication should either be reduced or stopped. When proper remedy has been taken, the patient will be recovered shortly.

III: serious toxin reaction.

IV: death.

Once again, "When chemotherapy fails, natural medicines must usher in." said Chairman Schmitt of the International Cancer Treatment League.

Therefore, the whole world is expecting from natural medicines. Except for a few of them, most herbal medications are free from radical side effects and they help stabilize the body's condition. China No. 1 Tian Xian Liquid, is made from natural raw ingredients which cause no side effects. The US Cancer Center has also proven that it does not contain acute toxins.

According to China No. 1 Tian Xian Capsule development project, the results of a clinical test shown in Table 5 is that one third of patients have 1 to 11 toxic reactions including slight digestive organ disorders, uneasiness, and vomiting. However, when the same test was performed using the liquid form, the result was almost zero.

The toxin reaction tests done according to immunology and pathology guidelines show that the China No. 1 Tian Xian Liquid does not produce the same side effects on blood, heart, liver, neurological system, hair and skin as radiation and chemotherapy do.

RELIEVING SIDE EFFECTS FROM RADIOTHERAPY AND CHEMOTHERAPY

The fact that the China No. 1 Tian Xian Liquid suppresses the side effects of radiation therapy and chemotherapy was proven by clinical tests. The side effects of radiation therapy are shown in Table 6. A relief from these side effects will mean a reduction of physical and mental suffering.

When the oral cavity ulcer and vomiting disappear, a patient will regain his appetite and of course his energy. In addition, when the loss of white blood cell, red blood cell, platelet and hemoglobin is under control, immunity improves. In other words, if these negative side effects are controlled, the quality of life and chances for survival for these cancer patients will greatly improve.

Improvements in the quality of life are the most important aspects of successful cancer treatments. Whether or not the physical and mental pain are reduced, the natural cure of cancer is still an issue.

Cancer is a disease that drains human energy. Cancer cells take away the body nutrition and sometimes cause great pain and consume a great deal of energy due to increasing pressure, subsequently reducing immunity. Furthermore, the side effects of radiation therapy and chemotherapy drain the rest of the body's energy which deprives it to be replenished.

Side effects cause great pain and anxiety, therefore, we must try to help patients alleviate the pain and give them courage and moral support to combat cancer.

REVEALING THE ANTI CANCER PROPERTIES AND EFFECTS OF CHINA NO. 1 TIAN XIAN LIQUID

To date, over 400,000 cancer patients in more than 20 countries are using China No. 1 Tian Xian Liquid. A survey conducted by the International Rehabilitation of Cancer Association (Hong Kong Headquarters), shows that over 80% of users expressed their confidence in the medicine. The figure is identical to the clinical tests done by China and US Cancer Center-an effective rate over 80%.

Now, let's see how China No. 1 Tian Xian Liquid functions. (i..e., how it suppresses cancer cell from multiplying, produces energy to combat cancer, improves immunity and subsequently cures cancer.)

Table 6: Comparison of Side Effect between Radiotherapy and China
No. 1 Tian Xian Liquid

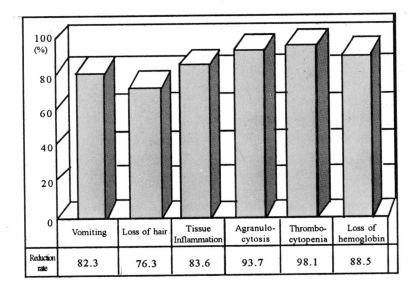

	Vomiting	Loss of hair	Tissue Inflammation	Agranulo-cytosis	Thrombo-cytopenia	Loss of hemoglobin
Reduction rate	82.3	76.3	83.6	93.7	98.1	88.5

In July of 1998, I was invited to give a speech at the 4th Japan International Cancer Convention organized by the US Cancer Control Association-Japan Branch. The aim of the convention is to share the results of using Chinese medicine either singly or in combination with Western medical treatment of cancer treatment.

My subject was the Study on the Anti Cancer Effects of China No. 1 Tian Xian Liquid-Natural Raw Medicines from China. In my report, clinical test results were also given. The most striking characteristics of China No. 1 Tian Xian Liquid are its ability to promote self-curing and its maximum natural curing ability.

At the same time, it suppresses cancer cells, slow the spread of cancer cells, relieves pain and improves immunity.

After six months of editing the content of my speech, it finally appeared in the documented version that I have given the highlights of my accomplishments in research. Since its contents are very technical, I will only mention the functions and effects of China No. 1 Tian Xian Liquid here.

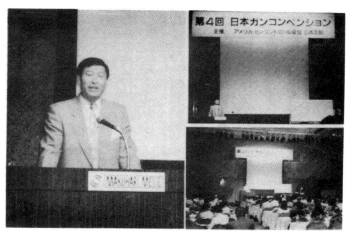

80   *Author delivering a speech at the 4th japan Cancer International Conference*

First, the major anti cancer function of China No. 1 Tian Xian Liquid is shown in Table 7.

1. Blocking cancer cells

2. Adjusting metabolism

3. Improving immunity

4. Micro element effect

Here are the description of 1 through 4.

Table 7: Major Anti cancer Functions and Effects of China No. 1 Tian Xian Liquid

1.	**Blocking cancer cells** The contents of China No.1 Tian Xian Liquid block the growth and multiplication of cancer cells.
(1)	To block the multiplicity of cancer cells at a certain stage and thereby kill them.
(2)	to stop cancer cells breathing at the stage of metabolism.
(3)	To damage cancer cells and let them dissolve. **[raw medicines that block cancer cells growth]** Rhizoma Arisaematis, Rhizoma Curcumae, Radix Aconiti, Radix Auklandiae, Radix Scrophulariae, Resina Garciniae, Sophora Alopecuroides, Herba Rabdosiae Rubescentis.
2.	**Adjusting metabolism** To change all kinds of metabolisms that cancer cells require and thereby suppress their multiplication. To improve the body invaded by cancer cells, to improve immunity against cancer cells, and thereby suppress the multiplication of cancer cells. **[raw medicines that adjust metabolism]** Black Nightshade, Solanum Lyratum Thunb, Herba Sarcandrae, Radix Angelicae, Sincensis, Radix Salviae Miltiorrhizae, tulip.
3.	**Improving immunity** To suppress cancer cell multiplication and to produce immunity, to control change in environment, and to promote killer cell activities. **[raw medicines that improves immunity]** Radix Rehmanniae, fungi, Radix Acantheopanacis Sentikcosi, Radix Astragali, Ginseng, Poria Polysaccharide, Ginsen Soapgenin, Radix Astra gali Polysaccharide, Radix Trichosanthis.

1. Blocking cancer cells. During the growth of cancer cells, we block them at a certain stage of development to repress multiplicity. A cell needs many elements during separation and multiplication to proceed DNA composition, RNA composition, and protein composition. If we can only stop cancer cells from multiplying in a certain way to suppress its spread. The raw medicines performing this function are shown in Table 7. However, not all raw medicines listed in the table are selected for China No. 1 Tian Xian Liquid. In the selection of raw medicines, we have adopted a more stringent set of criteria for choosing suitable ingredients.

2. Adjusting metabolism. Simply speaking, we use raw medicines to produce a hostile environment where cancer cells cannot easily multiply.

3. Improving immunity. There are various immune mechanisms in the human body. We are trying to stimulate them to resist cancer. While helping T-cells and B-cells suppress cancer cells, we improve the body immunity through the interference system.

4. Micro element effects. The micro element effect was mentioned in the previous chapter. All raw medicines used in China No. 1 Tian Xian Liquid are from Changbai Mountain and are rich in selenium, which is

responsible for preventing cancer cells from splitting but also in suppressing the growth and spread of tumors.

The anti cancer functions and effects of China No. 1 Tian Xian Liquid are presented on page 72. It is effective in blocking cancer cell growth, adjusting metabolism, improving immunity, and pushing cancer gene elements. When properly prescribed, raw medicines will produce extra effects to combat cancer.

RELIEVING SIDE-EFFECTS AND TREATING TERMINAL CANCER

Now we will give clinical reports to demonstrate the effects of China No. 1 Tian Xian Liquid on various cancers. China No. 1 Tian Xian Liquid cures symptoms of middle and terminal stage cancers, including difficulty in swallowing and severe pain. In addition, it also relieves the side effects brought about by radiotherapy and chemotherapy. The side effects are shown in Table 6.

Therefore, the severe pain experienced by patients from terminal cancer is one of the most important symptoms to suppress. When pain seeps in, vital energy is lost, and one's courage is diminished.

Table 8 shows the effect of China No. 1 Tian Xian Liquid on esophagus and stomach of terminal cancer patients. Notice especially the total improvement of very stable patients, which is as high as 97.5%. The key to relieving pain is suppress first then the multiplicity and transfer of cancer cells is deterred. As a result, pain will disappear.

Table 8: Relief Effect of China No. 1 Tian Xian Liquid
on Terminal Esophagus and Stomach Cancers

	Swallow Difficulty	Pain	Loss of Appetite
Subjects (82)	-	-	-
Improved	66.2%	59.6%	57.3%
Very Stable	29.7%	37.9%	38.4%
Increasingly Serious	4.1%	2.5%	4.3%

Furthermore, China No.1 Tian Xian Liquid has special effect on treating difficulty in swallowing (95.9) and loss of appetite (95.9%) and loss of appetite (95.7) for esophagus and stomach cancer. Once pain disappears, the patient can eat again so that energy levels increase, bodily functions resumes, immunity improves, and the courage to combat cancer is strengthened.

Therefore, when China No. 1 Tian Xian Liquid is used in combination with radiation therapy and chemotherapy, it can relieve the side effects and thereby cure cancer. The combined use of China No. 1 Tian Xian Liquid with radiotherapy and chemotherapy is discussed in Chapter 4.

EXPERIMENTS SHOW THAT NATURAL CHINESE MEDICINE MAKES CANCER DISAPPEAR

Now I would like to tell you about some examination and clinical results. They show how China No. 1 Tian Xian Liquid works on cancer cells.

The effect on cancer cells is shown on the pictures on p.86. The upper one is taken before the use of China No. 1 Tian Xian Liquid, and the lower one shows the cancer cells after using China No. 1 Tian Xian for a month. It is clear that the number of white blood cells increases around the cells and how they kill cancer cells after improvement in immunity.

Pictures on **p. 87** show the condition of lung and esophagus cancers after using China No. 1 Tian Xian Liquid.

A 3 x 4 cm tumor was found in left lung from the x-ray examination of Ms Ju Yuh Lan. After using China No. 1 Tian Xian Liquid for over two months, x-rays show that the tumor almost disappeared.

A 10cm tumor was found in the esophagus in the x-ray examination of Ms. Ding Shwu Ing and she could not swallow. After using China No. 1 Tian Xian Liquid for 3 months, the tumor was reduced to approximately 4cm.

The patients brought pictures of x-ray pictures.

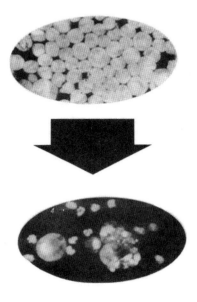

Cancer cells before using China No. 1 Tian Xian Liquid (upper). After using China No. 1 Tian Xian Liquid for one month, the number of white blood cells increased. It proves that cancer cells have been removed (lower).

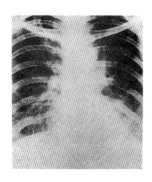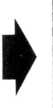

Lung Cancer - Ms. Ju before treatment.

X-ray examination after 12 months shows that the tumor almost disappears.

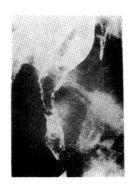

Esophagus Cancer - Ms. Ding before treatment.

X-ray examination after 3 months shows that the tumor reduces.

CHAPTER
5

TO IMPROVE THE EFFICIENCY OF OPERATION, RADIOTHERAPY AND CHEMOTHERAPY

CHINA NO. 1 TIAN XIAN LIQUID INCREASES ITS EFFICIENCY WHEN USED WITH OTHER TREATMENTS AND REMOVES LOSS OF APPETITE, UNEASINESS AND DIARRHEA.

MIXED TREATMENT HAS BEEN USED IN CANCER TREATMENT TO IMPROVE EFFICIENCY

WHEN ONE talks about cancer, almost everyone considers it as an incurable disease. However, following the advancement of Western medicine and technology, great advancements have been made in cancer treatment.

With the advent of medical technology, new advancement in operative techniques have come to the fore in cancer operation and surgery. With the combined use of radiotherapy and chemotherapy integrated with other holistic therapies, the over all treatment has greatly produced astonishing results. These results lend a better chance for cancer patients to survive.

However, no one can deny that there is still no absolute treatment for cancer using Western approach. The limits have been mentioned in previous chapters and here is a detailed description of these problems.

Scientific is good to describe cancer treatment using Western medicine. As a researcher of Western medicine, the present status of their cancer treatment has been long recognized without dynamism though, but they have merits to consider. But if we go by statistics, how many cancer patients treated with Western modalities of healing have been cured? And for how long have these cancer patients survived?

In Western medicine of cancer treatment, the doctors usually identify the source of cancer with one option, to remove by surgery. This approach will create traumatic impact to the human body.

Operation refers to the removal of the source or the affected area of cancer and it is very effective in cases during preliminary stages of cancer. However, the spread of cancer can never be predicted so that operations performed in patients during the middle stage are no longer effective.

Radiation therapy refers to the use of radiation to kill cancer cells and is the same principle used in chemotherapy. However, no matter what method is used, it is impossible to kill all the cancer cells. For normal cells are killed at the same time and produce drastic side effects. Because of the pain brought by the side effects, the patients suffer more.

Operations result in an increasing number of health problems.

Western medicine has just began to embrace the holistic belief that adjusting the body's condition, improving its immunity, supplementing its energy and stimulating its natural defenses are the most important ways of improving cancer treatment.

This is the reason why Holistic Medicine emerged. This approach revolves around the mind, body, emotions and spirit of every individual as a collective unit. Integrated approach of various modalities of healing are employed from Western Medicine to Traditional Chinese Medicine, from psychoneuro approach to mystical approach.

CHINESE MEDICINE - KEY TO HOLISTIC MEDICINE

Holistic medicine is not a new concept anymore. In the first chapter, we have discussed its ramifications. Since 1930's, it has been developed and many countries followed suit. The British Cancer Clinic in the United Kingdom offers complementary medicines such as homeopathy, body therapies and other holistic approaches. This was supported by HRH Prince Charles. Other countries like Germany, Switzerland and Japan have created holistic groups to include integrative medicine in their therapeutic practices.

A Japanese investigation team visited the Changbai Mountain Pharmacology Research Institute.

Director Obitsu Ryoichi of the Obitsu Sankei Hospital is a famous doctor who has used holistic medicine to treat cancer in recent times. He is also the Chair of the association.

It was 10 years ago when I met Obitsu-Ryoichi just after I have developed China No. 1 Tian Xian Capsule. He was so interested in Chinese medicine that he personally visited China. After that, we met several times in international conferences held in Japan and elsewhere. He was the first doctor I know who was active in holistic medicine and I admired him most.

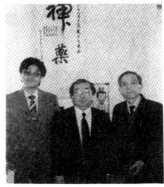

Director Obitsu Ryoichi (center) and the author in China

91

The medical ideas of Japan's Holistic Medicine Association are as follows:

1. Holistic health is the cornerstone.
2. Natural cure is the start
3. Patients get cured naturally and thus help others.
4. Collective treatments
5. Self-realization of full attention to disease.

It is undeniable that China No. 1 Tian Xian Liquid has proven many beneficial effects.

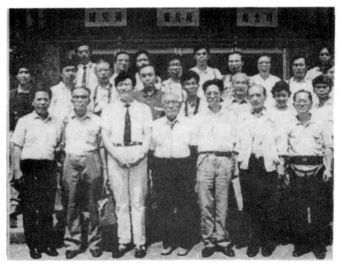

Picture of Japanese visitors at Chang Bani Shan Institute of Medicine

A MULTIDIMENSIONAL, MIXED TREATMENT WILL HELP IMPROVE THE EFFECT OF TREATMENT

Holistic medicine has been the only approach in cancer treatment I have admired for a long time. I have always believed that there must be more than one method to cure cancer. As there are many different methods to fight cancer (Chapters I & II), I hope readers will find out more about holistic medicine in the first two chapters

Much emphasis has been put on Western medicine. When different therapies are combined in a treatment program, the effect will be increased.

First of all, I advise patients to have operations when cancer is detected during initial stages, however, I suggest using the China No. 1 Tian Xian Liquid to prevent metastasis and recurrence of cancer, whether a patient has undergone an operation or has received radiotherapy or chemotherapy. One can prevent subsequent growth and recurrence of cancer by using the China No. 1 Tian Xian Liquid at the same time for three months then reducing the standard dose for six months.

Operation will fail in most cases during middle and terminal stages of cancer. Even if an operation is undergone, metastasis and recurrence are unavoidable. From my point of view, when China No. 1 Tian Xian Liquid is used in combination with radiation therapy or chemotherapy, it can help relieve the side effects and can improve the efficacies of therapies. These truths have been identified in various clinical reports.

For terminal cancer cases deemed incurable especially when radiotherapy and chemotherapy fail, holistic medicine combined with Traditional Chinese Medicine can offer a higher batting average for survival.

I am stating the truth, the beneficial effect of China No. 1 Tian Xian Liquid on terminal cancer is undeniable.

"Why is Chinese medicine effective against cancer?" This is the question usually posed by practitioners of Western medicine. What properties do Chinese herbal medicines have that they are enigmatically efficacious in curing cancer. The Western medicine people are awed by the tremendous effects of Traditional Chinese Medicine even sometimes they lack scientific validation.

However, the 3000 year old Chinese medicine will take a very long time to verify.

Holistic medicine, Chinese medication, intensive research and anything useful for my research in curing cancer became my ultimate consideration. We need to consider every holistic and therapeutic approach to effectively cure cancer patients.

Of course, Western medicine is still recognized as the forefront of cancer treatment. If Western medicine fails, holistic medicine is a veritable option. We should give hope to cancer patients who have lost chance for survival and use every holistic therapy there is to keep them alive.

COMBINED USE WITH OPERATIONS, RADIOTHERAPY AND CHEMO-THERAPY TO OVERCOME CANCER

Here is a description of a few successful cases of China No. 1 Tian Xian Liquid used in combination with Western medicine treatments. The first case is an esophagus tumor at 10cm.

The operation was exceptionally difficult. The patient had received radiation and chemotherapy and he suffered severe pain. He came to my clinic when nobody could do anything more for him.

After reading his diagnostic record and examining his condition, I prescribed him heavy dosage of China No. 1 Tian Xian Liquid, 80 CC daily, which was doubled up from the normal dose. I advised him to use the liquid for one week and 12 capsules a day for 3 weeks. The normal dose is 40 CC liquid and 8 capsules a day.

In the beginning, it was difficult for him to swallow during the first three days of treatment. On the fourth day, he could smoothly ingest the medication. A week later, he began to use China No. 1 Tian Xian Capsule and three weeks later, he began eating liquid food. In a month's time, the side effects were gone and he began to eat congee and similar soft diet.

Three months later, he had an x-ray examination which showed that the tumor had reduced in size.

In this case, it is difficult to tell whether it is the radiation therapy and chemotherapy or the China No. 1 Tian Xian Liquid and capsule which brought cure. In short, the difficulty in swallowing was relieved and I think that is the most important initial part in combating cancer.

The next case shows a spread of cancer from colon to liver. There is a 1.4 x 1.2cm tumor on the left side of the liver, and it was diagnosed as liver cancer. The chance of success was extremely low. Even the doctor ruled out operation and began radiotherapy and chemotherapy. The patient's daughter was about to get married and he wondered if he would still be alive to join them. He came to my clinic in great pain.

I immediately prescribed China No. 1 Tian Xian Pill No. 6 and China No. 1 Tian Xian Liquid. The dose of the liquid was doubled from the regular, and the capsule was 1.5 times greater I recommended that he uses the prescription for 1 month.

The tumor became smaller after a month and almost disappeared in two months. Both therapies have been used and both deserve the credit. However, we are positive that combined treatment was effective.

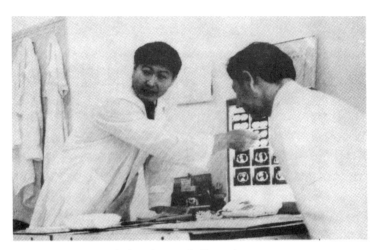

Author observes the X-ray diagnosis

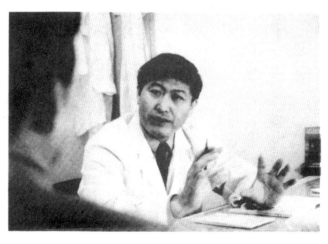

Author gives prescription to the patient.

CLINICAL RESULTS OF COMBINED USED WITH RADIOTHERAPY AND CHEMOTHERAPY

A multidimensional, mixed cancer treatment refers to the combined use of radiotherapy, chemotherapy and China No. 1 Tian Xian Liquid. Clinical tests show that the result of such treatment is exceptionally efficient and effective. That is why China No. 1 Tian Xian Liquid has drawn so much attention in Western medicine.

In other words, it helps prevent metastasis and recurrence of cancer, relieve side effects of radiation therapy and chemotherapy and suppress cancer cell growth. It improves immunity and the natural defenses (macrophages) of the human body, accelerates rate of recovery and prolongs lives of terminal cancer patients.

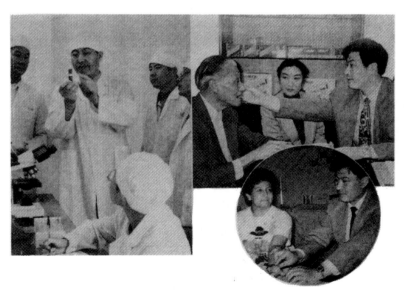

Researchers of the institute and author (center). Author goes to patients all over the world.

The comparison of using radiotherapy and chemotherapy alone and in combination with China No. 1 Tian Xian Liquid is shown in Table 9.

The result in the upper table shows that when radiotherapy is used in combination with China No. 1 Tian Xian Liquid, the cure rate i.e., disappearance of tumor, is double for the therapy alone.

From the table at the bottom, it is clear that the rate of case by chemotherapy alone is 3.6%, it is 29.2% while used in combination with China No. 1 Tian Xian Liquid. Either cured or with striking relief of 12% greater, the assured effective rate is 20%.

Table 9: Clinical comparison of using radiotherapy and chemotherapy alone and in combination with China No. 1 Tian Xian Liquid.

(Comparison of using radiotherapy alone and in combination with China No. 1 Tian Xian Liquid)

Effect Group	Subjects	Cured	Striking Effect	Effective	Ineffective	Relief	Effective
Combined Use	20	13	6	1	0	19	20
		65%	30%	5%	0%	95%	100%
Radiation Therapy Alone	20	6	6	8	0	12	20
		30%	30%	40%	0%	60%	100%

* China No. 1 Tian Xian Liquid 1350 ml + full rate radiation DT6000cgy-7500cgy and full rate radiation alone DT6000cgy-7500cgy (approx. P=0.01)

(Comparison of using chemotherapy alone and in combination with China No. 1 Tian Xian Liquid)

Effect Group	Subjects	Cured	Striking Effect	Effective	Ineffective	Relief	Effective
Combined Use	48	14	12	12	10	26	38
		29.2%	25%	25%	20.8%	54.2%	79.2%
Chemotherapy Alone	56	2	22	8	24	24	32
		3.6%	39.20%	40%	14.3%	2.9%	57.2%

CHAPTER 6

THE AMAZING DEVELOPMENT OF THE WORLD-RENOWNED NATURAL CHINA NO. 1 TIAN XIAN LIQUID

SCIENTIFICALLY VERIFIED BY THE US-BRI IN A RESEARCH PAPER

RESEARCH ACHIEVEMENTS ANNOUNCED AT JAPAN AND U.S. INTERNATIONAL CONVENTIONS

IN JULY of 1998, I was invited to deliver a speech at the 4th International Cancer Convention in Japan held in Shinkoko Conference Center, Chiba, Japan.

Here is an introduction to the nature of the convention experts who took part in the convention.

The topic of the convention was "Cancer-Possibility of Survival" through substitute treatment and holistic treatment to demonstrate the great survival power of human beings. Experts from world wide came to share their achievements in cancer treatment.

Participants included the holistic treatment inventor Dr. Obitsu Ryoichi, Dr. Higashiyama Akinori who combines natural treatments with Western medicine; Dr. Carl Simon who adopts psycho-treatment in cancer treatment and Dr. Gary G. Gordon, who advocates metabolic treatment.

The topic of my paper was 'Anti Cancer Functions of China No. 1 Tian Xian Liquid'- A viewpoint on Cancer from Chinese medicine. It was an account for the cancer treatment using Chinese medicine and clinical reports about China No. 1 Tian Xian Liquid.

It was the second time I gave a speech at the US Cancer Control Association-Japan Chapter. It is very important to exchange knowledge with experts worldwide and I have mentioned part of my speech in previous chapter.

Later in October of 1998, I gave two more speeches on the same topic in Los Angeles and San Francisco.

Such opportunities did not only broadened my views but also enabled me to make progress through the exchange of information with other experts.

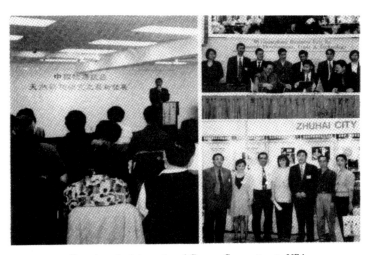

Speech at the International Cancer Convention in USA

CHINA No. 1 TIAN XIAN LIQUID DRAWS ATTENTION OF U.S BRI RESEARCH TEAM

My speech drew the attention of R. W. Bradford, Director of the US-BRI Institute who showed great interest in China No. 1 Tian Xian Liquid.

Dr. Bradford established the FRC Biomedicine Research Institute in Taiwan and the Bradford Medical Clinic. He is the director of both. In these establishments, they study cancer treatment and the treatment of other chronic diseases through Western medicine.

He is a pioneer and authority in active enzyme research and he believes that all diseases are related to the change of enzymes in human body. Since the details are technical and specific, I shall omit them. Simply speaking, Dr. Bradford uses a unique method to calculate the quantity of enzymes in the human body to diagnose the disease and health condition of a patient. Then, he watches the blood in a slide under a special microscope to analyze condition of the disease.

According to his theory, active enzymes are the causes of cancer and other diseases. It is due to the overreaction of enzyme activity when air enters our body. Originally, enzymes serve to protect the human body.

Why are active enzymes the cause of diseases? It is a problem that the body produces more than what is needed. The causes of cancer complications include chronic stimulation and mutation. Active enzymes exist in both cases. Moreover, when an active enzyme combines with unsaturated fat it produces excessive acidic fat. It can be the real cause of all kinds of chronic diseases.

Dr. Bradford and his team widely applied this theory in diagnosis and treatment. In the course of studying active enzymes, his team discovered this theory can be applied in both diagnosis and treatment. In the course of studying active enzymes, they discovered the importance. Chinese raw medicines and China No. 1 Tian Xian Liquid. Because most members of the team are Chinese, they have greater interest in Chinese medicine and raw medicines.

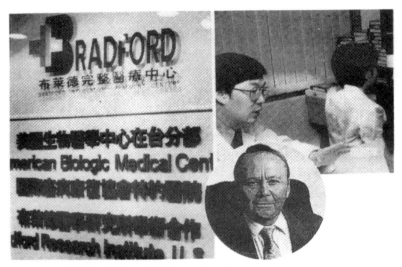

US-BRI Institute and FRC Biomedicine Research Institute.

RESEARCH REPORTS ON THE WORLD RENOWED CHINA NO. 1 TIAN XIAN LIQUID

Research on China No. 1 Tian Xian Liquid and its effects on oncogene and acidic fat. The project was conducted by Dr. Bradford and several international specialists of different research institutions.

Researchers included doctors from the China Tumor Society, professors from Biophysics Institute of the China Research Institute of Science, clinical biochemistry doctors from Cleveland University and researchers from the Combined Health Medicine of Capital University. The project lasted for 2 years, and the reports were published in both Chinese and English. The paper is concise and powerful, and it is very valuable especially for me. However, since the contents are very technical and difficult to understand. I shall briefly describe the framework.

1. Toxic tests and researches of China No. 1 Tian Xian Liquid.
2. Research on the anti cancer functions of China No. 1 Tian Xian Liquid on implanted tumor S180 and liver cancer.
3. Empirical research on the impact of non-specific immune func tion brought by China No. 1 Tian Xian Liquid to guinea pigs.
4. Empirical research on the oncogene and acidic fat removal function of China No. 1 Tian Xian Liquid.

Deputy Director Ding Ke Xiang of China Tumor Society draws the following conclusions about China No. 1 Tian Xian Liquid's functions on tumor.

The results show that FRC 1 (Improved China No. 1 Tian Xian Liquid) has a striking effect on tumor S180 and liver cancer.

1. China No. 1 Tian Xian Liquid helps activate bruises, remove

body heat and poisonous substance, remove spit, supplement energy and blood. In the case of liver cancer, it helps strengthen the good and eliminate the bad and to remove the true cause of the disease.

2. The Chinese medicine used in China No. 1 Tian Xian Liquid helps produce good substances for human body, promotes health and digestion. It also helps regulate breathing, remove excretion, improve circulation, make blood and other immune functions. Some of our body functions also help accomplish similar things, and it can suppress the growth of tumor.

3. The contents of China No. 1 Tian Xian Liquid help regulate human immunity, strengthen the function of the internal skin system network, and suppress the growth of tumor.

4. The contents of China No. 1 Tian Xian Liquid helps to sup press the DNA metabolism, RNA, and DNA combination of cancer cells, thereby killing cancer cells.

5. China No. 1 Tian Xian Liquid helps to remove the oncogene; it is a critical cancer-trigger agent which China No. 1 Tian Xian Liquid suppresses.

The growth, progression and suppression of tumor is a complex biological process. The mechanical research of the individual functions rely on future empirical studies.

According to Dr. Bradford, Dr. CHIU Zhong-feng who drew the following conclusions on the anti-oxidation function in direct treatment of China No. 1 Tian Xian Liquid.

"There is no direct evidence to indicate how China No. 1 Tian Xian Liquid kills cancer cells and it is our future task to find out how it works.

According to our research, we are sure of the following three complex functions and further proof has been obtained."

First, it reduces the active oxidative activity. According to the high anti acid activity, we have observed the quantity of active oxygen and oxidized fat in preliminary stage cancer patients. The quantity of both reduces when the tumor gets smaller.

Second, it improves human immunity and promotes healing. If the immune system is not revived, no disease can be healed, and that is the result in our experiment.

Third, it helps suppress the activation of cancer cells. So far, we still don't know how it did it, but the result is real.

In the general conclusion of the research, Dr. Bradford says, 'I give my highest esteem to China No. 1 Tian Xian Liquid. although we are unsure' what in the medication did it. It does suppress the multiplicity, transfer and recurrence of cancer cells and relieves the side effects brought about by Western medical treatment.'

'When I learned of the result, I realized my great contribution to cancer treatment. It is simple to use, either as liquid or in capsule form. It suppresses side effects and kills cancer cell and subsequently brings back patients of course. Of course, China No. 1 Tian Xian Liquid itself does not cause any side effects and it is wonderful to know the effect of cancer medication at all stages has been proven already by Western medicine.'

'In summary, I believe the development of China No. 1 Tian Xian Liquid has changed the view on cancer treatment. From the viewpoint of alternative medicine such as this, we can provide hope of survival to every cancer patient. Herbal medicines have proven their efficacy in oncological cases. Cancer now can be cured and this school of thought has greatly contributed to the thinking of Western medicine.

THE BEGINNING OF MODIFYING CHINA NO. 1 TIAN XIAN LIQUID

China No. 1 Tian Xian Capsule is the mother of China No. 1 Tian Xian Liquid. In 1995, the Improved China No. 1 Tian Xian Liquid came out more strengthened and improved. My reason why I keep on improving the product is to save people. This is my foremost duty and mission in life.

For instance, during the liquefaction of China No. 1 Tian Xian Capsule we discovered that even the quality of raw materials has improved their effect but only fresh ingredients were used. Then we kept on trying new combination to come up with new formula in order to strengthen its effects in order to produce the most effective anti cancer medicine.

Of course, even the China No. 1 Tian Xian Capsule was not the final product. It has undergone five stages, Nos. 1, 3, 5, 6 and 7. Please refer to Table 10 for details.

China No. 1 Tian Xian Capsule is an auxiliary to the China No. 1 Tian Xian Liquid. China No. 1 Tian Xian Liquid has solved the disadvantages of capsule such as difficulty in swallowing and stomach pain.

Now the suppository form of China No. 1 Tian Xian product has been developed. Suppositories can help shorten lead-time to absorption, therefore it is best for seriously ill patients. In addition, plaster form China No. 1 Tian Xian product also appears to relieve the severe pain of patients who suffer from stomach, esophagus, respiratory tract, thyroid and liver cancers. In summary, the combined use of China No. 1 Tian Xian Liquid and other forms of China No. 1 Tian Xian products can double the original positive effects.

In my opinion, the more modalities of treatment, the better the results.

Although the liquid is given in small quantities, it helps tremendously, spiritually and physically. In fact, according to my clinical research on raw medicine dripping, the result is beyond our imagination.

There are two reasons why we have changed the package of China No. 1 Tian Xian Liquid in December of 1998.

First, there are too many counterfeits in Hong Kong, Taiwan, China and Southeast Asia exporting to Japan, damaging the credibility of the authentic product. To distinguish counterfeits and similar products, we have changed the package.

Second, we have improved the bottle. Food grade plastic material has been used to strengthen the quality and to avoid damage during transport. The same material has been used for both the bottle and the cover and it is now easier to open.

China No. 1 Tian Xian Liquid has passed the UPC international bar code permit in USA in May 1998 to become a global product. The US Food and Drug Authority considers it as a dietary supplement (document LI 149534 in approving the product).

Table 10: Major Raw Medicines and Effects of China No. 1 Tian Xian Capsule

	China No. 1 Tian Xian Capsule	Effect	Application
No. 1	Radix Trichosanthis, Semen Impatientis, Venenum Bufonis, Black Nightshade, Radix Astragali, Ginsen, Calculus Bovis, Polyporus Umbellata, Hedyotis Didduse Wild, Clematis Root.	Remove body heat and poisonous substance; Supplement energy and blood, combined use	Esophagus cancer, Stomach cancer, Intestinal cancer, Digestion system with radiation therapy cancers. and chemotherapy
No. 3	Radix Astragali, Ginsen Radix Ophiopogonis, Fructus Jujubae, Rhizoma atractylodis Macrocephalae, Fructus Schisandrae, Indigo Naturalis Radix Rehmanniae, Radix Angelicae Sincensis, Radix Glycyrrhizae	Supplement energy and blood, strengthen spleen and stomach, remove body heat and poisonous substance, improve immunity.	Relieve side effects of radiotherapy and chemotherapy leukemia
No. 5	Arisaema Erubescens, Fritillaria Cirrhosa Ginsen, Radix Astragali, Asparagus Lucidus Lindl, Cortex Magnoliae Officinalis, Herba Houtuyniae, Herba Scutellariae Ba Rbatae, Rhizoma Brain tumor.	Good to breath and lung, remove phlegm, suppress pain, remove body heat, avoid blood vomiting. Laryngeal cancer,	Lung cancer, Oral cavity cancer, Nasopharyngeal passage cancer, Pinelliae, Radix Glycyrrhizae.
No. 6	Calculus Bovis, Hebra Artenisiae Scopariae, Radix Bupleuri, Radix Auklandiae, Radix Curcumae, Rhizoma Corydalis, Rhizoma Spargani, Rhizoma Curcumae, Ginsen, Polyporus Umbellata	Remove body heat and poisonous substance, remove swollen muscle, promote blood circulation and suppress pain.	Liver cancer, Gall bladder cancer Spleen cancer, Cirrhosis of liver, Chronic hapatitis.
No. 7	Scolopendra, Scorpio, Cornu Cervi, Nidus Vespae, Ginsen, Radix Astragali, Fructus Trichosanthis, Spica Prunellae Pseudobulbus Cremastrae Pleiones.	Supplement blood, promote blood circulation and suppress pain, improves benign tumor	Breast cancer, Ovarian cancer, Cervial cancer, Thyroid cancer, Bone cancer, Testicular cancer Bladder cancer, Penis cancer Skin cancer

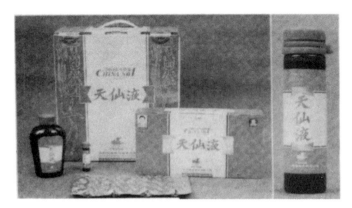

New packaging of China No. 1 Tian Xian Liquid starting December 1998

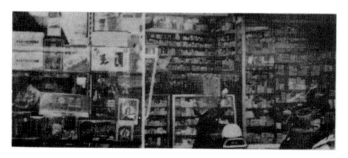

Drugstores in Hong Kong and Taiwan selling counterfeits of China No. 1 Tian Xian Liquid

THE NEW SUBJECT SEEKS THE ULTIMATE ANTI CANCER CHINESE
MEDICINE

Now I am engaged in research to produce the ultimate anti cancer
medicine. There are three main reasons:

1. To discover and to study raw medicines that have better anti
    cancer effects. So far, I have studied an average of 50 to 60 new
    raw medicines each year, I just want to find out the most effective
    ones in killing cancer cells.

2. To discover and study raw medicines that improve human im-
    munity. While surgery, radiotherapy and chemotherapy are still
    most widely accepted methods of cancer treatment, I must find
    out the most effective ones to relieve negative side effects and
    improve human immunity.

3. To discover and study raw medicines that can break cancer cells
    tissue and to disintegrate them from inside.

The next product will be the fortified China No. 1 Tian Xian
Liquid and clinical test started a year ago which showed that it
can prolong life of terminal cancer patients when surgery fails. Surprising
results have been found out when combined with radiotherapy and chemotherapy. There was no transfer of cancer cell and their damage rate rose,
healing rates increased by 20% and there was an efficacy rate of 90%. I
feel that the ultimate anti cancer Chinese medicine has entered a new
era.

People have long been viewing anti cancer Chinese medicine from
a critical Western viewpoint! They often question its effects. I frequently
ask myself. "Why China No. 1 Tian Xian Liquid?"

I found the answer in the long-term clinical tests. It has been ten
years now since the first China No. 1 Tian Xian medicines were devel-

oped. Over 400,000 patients have used it. We have received many thanks and great support. If it is ineffective, why are there so many people using it?

Before the invention of an anti cancer panacea and in time when cancer has become the No. 1 killer worldwide, I think the best way to prolong a patient's life will be better than just treating cancer. In other words, to help and encourage the patient to survive is more important than to find out why.

To discover ultimate anti cancer Chinese medicine will be my life-long mission. To look for a Chinese medicine that cures cancer in order to save lives will always be my objective.

2

WE CONQUER CANCER
WITH CHINESE NATURAL HERBAL MEDICINE

COMBATING CANCER WITH THE CHINESE NATURAL
HERBAL MEDICINE
CHINA NO. 1 TIAN XIAN LIQUID!
REPORTS FROM 50 PATIENTS WHO SUCCESSFULLY OVERCAME
CANCER WITH CHINA NO. 1 TIAN XIAN LIQUID.

True Voices from Recovered Cancer Patients Worldwide

In the beginning of this chapter, I would like to tell you the stories of patients who have overcome cancer using China No. 1 Tian Xian Liquid. They are patients from China, Japan, USA, Malaysia, Thailand, the Philippines, Hong Kong, and Taiwan.

Some travel great distances with their disease to tell me their stories, some sent me letters (as many as snowflakes), and some even extend their help, They tell the truth about China No. 1 Tian Xian Liquid-how it has saved their lives. Here are their voices.

These accounts are taken from my personal interviews and correspondences, cases from the International Rehabilitation of Cancer Association, Hong Kong global agent, China Japan Feida Union Co., Ltd. and Wang Zhen-Guo Office, International Rehabilitation of Cancer Association-Japan Branch.

Cancer is a global disease and unfortunately, the number of incurable cases keeps on rising. One should not, however, lose faith and courage in combating cancer. Hope and joy for survival are the keys to overcome them.

In this section, we are going to tell you how patients discovered China No. 1 Tian Xian Liquid, how they combated cancer and how they overcame it. With these stories, we hope to give you the courage and strength needed to fight and overcome cancer.

Unless authorized by the patient himself, all names mentioned in this section are fictitious. Due to printing limitations, some stories have been abridged.

Finally, we express our greatest gratitude to those who have shared their stories with us.

TRIUMPH OVER STOMACH CANCER

SIDE EFFECTS HAVE DISAPPEARED
MY STOMACH CONDITION IS GOOD AND HEALTHY
THROUGHOUT THE YEAR
Watase Nobuyuki (Age, 56, employee,
Saga City, Saga County, Japan)

SURGERY WAS conducted at the Social Security Hospital to remove about 75% of my stomach. I left the hospital about a week later. My daughter who was living in Tokyo returned to Saga to take care of me and she brought me a book about China No. 1 Tian Xian Liquid. I couldn't wait to finish the book before I wanted to try it so I bought some from importers. I began taking a dosage of 10ml, six times a day.

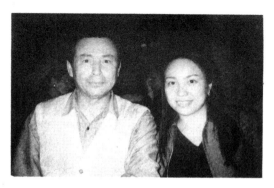

It's great to get rid of the side effects. Watase and his daughter.

According to the doctor, almost all patients would feel pain in the chest and sometimes would vomit after surgery. It's a normal reaction. After using China No. 1 Tian Xian Liquid, I did not feel anything. I weigh 85kg before the surgery to 65kg afterwards. However, I am back to 75kg a year later and then 80kg after three years. The abnormal size of my stomach returned to normal. My recovery astonished my doctor. After I regained my health, I returned to work as a volunteer firefighter.

I needed to inject medication once a week in combination with China No. 1 Tian Xian Liquid to maintain my immunity. I think it must be China No. 1 Tian Xian Liquid that relieved the side effects. The chief doctor told me that the cancer would possibly recur within 2 years. However, there was no sign of recurrence after three years. Even the follow-up quarterly examination did not show anything wrong. I regained my life.

Triumph Over Stomach Cancer

I recommend China No. 1 Tian Xian Liquid to
PATIENTS SUFFERING FROM DIGESTIVE SYSTEM CANCERS
Kijima Sakie (Age 79, from Tokyo, reported by her son)

THIS IS the story of my mother. She died eight months after the surgery. I just want to share my experience to all China No. 1 Tian Xian Liquid users.

When the doctor diagnosed my mother of stomach cancer, it had already spread to the intestine and spleen. The surgery is aimed at removing the entire stomach and major parts of her spleen and intestine especially all the infected tissues. After the surgery, relatives of my mother-in-law recommended China No. 1 Tian Xian Liquid to us. A month later, the nurse asked us out of curiosity, 'does it help to produce nutrition?' that was apparent in the case of my mother's rapid recovery. The consistent use of China No. 1 Tian Xian Liquid relieved the harsh side effects of chemotherapy.

After the surgery, an examination was done three months and showed that the tumor expanded. The doctor recommended the use of concentrated chemotherapy as last hope. The side effects would be extreme but the curative rate would be over 60%. To be or not to be, that was the question.

We accepted the suggestion and after a month's hospitalization, the side effects proved to be beyond our imagination which includes regurgitation and oral cavity inflammation. She could use China No. 1 Tian Xian Liquid for a month only. Why did we stop giving her China No. 1 Tian Xian Liquid? We will always regret it. When we gave her China No. 1 Tian Xian Liquid after coming home, it was too late. When she was sent to the hospital again, she never came home.

Even though my mother's case cannot prove anything about China No. 1 Tian Xian Liquid, it is through it that she recovered very fast. Her condition shows that China No. 1 Tian Xian Liquid did relieve the harsh side effects of chemotherapy.

However, when the concentrated chemotherapy is applied, side effects are always present. The suppository form of China No. 1 Tian Xian Liquid should have been used instead when she could not swallow anything.

I have tried many things, including shark's soft bone, water soluble kitosan, vitamin treatment, Agaliks horn, etc. China NO. 1 Tian Xian Liquid was the last one and it was the most effective one. A miracle did not come to my mother as I had wished. I recommend China No. 1 Tian Xian Liquid to digestive system cancer patients.

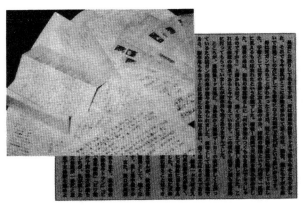

Letters from Japan and the letter of Kajima

TRIUMPH OVER STOMACH CANCER

FIRMLY BELIEVES OF THE MIRACLE THAT CHINA NO. 1 TIAN XIAN LIQUID BRINGS
Chen Min Zhao (Aged 60, retired soldier, Kaohsiung-Taiwan)

I WAS diagnosed of stomach cancer in June of 1998 and surgery was administered to remove my entire stomach. Since then, I suffered from abdominal pain and vomiting after eating. My wife told me that surgery was the only way to prevent cancer from spreading to other organs and throughout my whole body.

I left the hospital a month later. Upon learning China No. 1 Tian Xian Liquid from magazines, my wife immediately bought some books about the medicine and began reading them. I began to use China No. 1 Tian Xian Liquid in the beginning of August. When she learned of the particular effect of China No. 1 Tian Xian Liquid on stomach cancer, she brought it home immediately. At first. I was pessimistic about the medicine.

So I began to use China No. 1 Tian Xian Liquid. People said that it helps in improving immunity and recovering lost energy. I didn't believe it until I began to feel my body was recovering.

Everyone who visited me told me that I was getting better. I firmly believe that it was China No. 1 Tian Xian Liquid that brought me the miracle. I will continue to use it, until my cancer is gone.

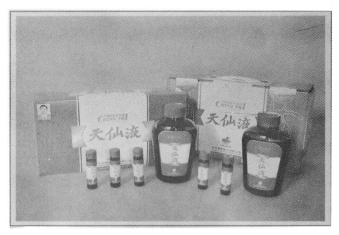

China No. 1 Tian Xian Liquid in new and improved packaging.

Triumph Over Stomach Cancer

Terminal patient diagnosed with less-than-one-month-to live still survives
Li Yu Xiang (aged 66, banking, Tseng City,
Guangdong, China)

My stomach has been very weak for a long time and I had a long history of digestive problems. In Autumn of 1990, I went to the hospital for an endoscopy examination of my stomach when my friend alerted me of my weight loss. The result showed that cancer had infected my esophagus and stomach and both of them were terminal.

They removed over 60% of my stomach during the first surgery. I felt very weak and fatigued afterwards. The excessive phlegm that I produced during the week following surgery annoyed me. Two weeks later, they told me that none of the treatments worked. I was forced to leave the hospital. I kept myself subjected to chemotherapy and I suffered all the typical side effects. My condition was very unstable, sometimes good and sometimes bad. I just decided to go to other hospitals. I was in a critical condition when I started to retain water in my lungs. I was transferred to Zhongshan Tumor Specialist Hospital in February. I was told that I had only a month to live. I don't want to die, I could not leave my children but I became very weak.

On January 21 of that year, I will never forget when my relatives recommended China No. 1 Tian Xian Liquid. I began getting better, I stopped using Western medicines.

It has been eight years now, I'm still using China No. 1 Tian Xian Liquid in smaller doses and there is no more sign of cancer. I survived.

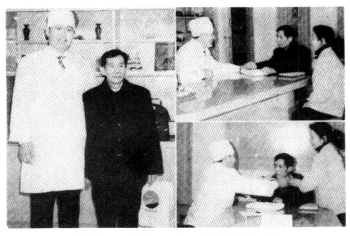

Mr. Wang-my lifesaver, the joyful Mr. & Mrs. Li

Triumph Over Stomach Cancer

Malignant tumor with a size of an egg disappears within a year
Yeung Ching Wan (Aged 58, housewife, HK)

It has been nine years now since I suffered from cancer. One day I passed out when I was working in a bank and an endoscopy examination showed that there was a tumor in my stomach.

'It was the size of a bean and made me feel like I had some kind of gastritis. Suddenly, it expanded like a wild horse to the size of an egg in less than a month. When cancer spreads this way, no surgery can save. I was told that I had no more than 3 months to live.'

This horrible news made everyone panic. My family tried to be calm and hide the truth. They told me that I might suffer from some kind of incurable disease. I did not want to die without knowing the truth so I asked the doctor. When he showed me the X-ray results he told me that I had only a month to live. I was so startled that I couldn't say a word. I decided not to have surgery or any type of therapy. I went home and wanted to spend my final days with my family.

I thought I might prolong or at least make my final days a little easier so I began using it. The vomiting and uneasiness went away and I regained my appetite. After using it continuously for a year, the once egg-size tumor shrank to the size of a bean. In an examination recently, the tumor totally disappeared.

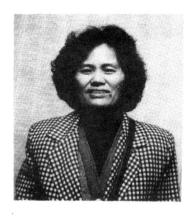

Friends recommend the China No. 1 Tian Xian Liquid and the tumor disappeared.

Triumph Over Stomach Cancer

Elderly People Should Avoid the Side Effect of Chemotherapy Kurosawa Kiku
(Aged 87, Ebetsu City-Hokkaido Japan, Reported by her daughter)

It was November of 1995 when my mother told me that she felt exceptionally tired when she woke up one morning. We went to a GP clinic and an endoscopy examination confirmed that her stomach cancer (CEA, mark 2.7) had recurred. To avoid the severe side effects of chemotherapy, she used Chinese medicine but the effect was unsatisfactory.

In February of 1996, my son brought home some China No. 1 Tian Xian Liquid from Taiwan. It is very famous in Taiwan so I gave my mother four bottles a day. It was surprising that the mark reduces to 2.0 after using it for just a month. In May, the mark fell to 1.6 and kept going down. In August, the miraculous medicine cured my mother. She stopped using it then. In October, she was infected by unknown acute intestinal inflammation which caused fever to rise at 40 °C and diarrhea for three consecutive days. After hospitalization for three months, she went home but the diarrhea started again and the mark rose to 2.7.

In January of 1997, I started giving her three bottles of China No. 1 Tian Xian Liquid per day. By October, the mark had fallen to 1.4

and the condition remained stable. Then I reduced her intake to a bottle per day. Now she feels no pain. Although she is weak, she has good appetite. She began to lose her memory and difficulty in sleeping as elderly people do. For me, to be free from annoyances are luxuries of life.

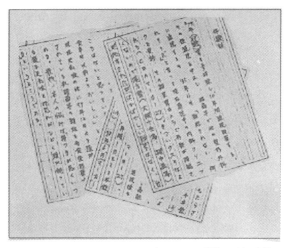

Letters from the son tellling the information of China No. I Tian Xian Liquid

TRIUMPH OVER INTESTINAL CANCER

PATIENTS WITH WIDE SPREAD COMPLEX CANCERS ARE
ABLE TO LEAVE THE HOSPITAL
Ooshima Kouichi (Aged 62, Kashiwa Shi, Chiba, Japan)

IN DECEMBER of 1997, I was told that I am suffering from portal hepatitis bile duct cancer and upper rectum cancer. They administered drainage treatment immediately. Surgery for the bile duct was impossible so I tried chemotherapy but it was in vain. The doctor then told me that I could only try radiotherapy. So I went to another hospital to receive ra

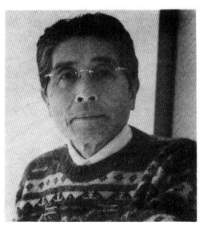

My family send me the tape of Mr Wang's speech and I decided to use it after listening to it.

131

diotherapy in January. In April, I had surgery for my rectum cancer and in May, they stopped the drainage treatment. Then I went home and in two weeks, I had to return to the hospital for another drainage treatment.

During that time, I began using China No. 1 Tian Xian Liquid regularly. I learned about it in a book and pamphlets given by a friend. I started using it on a trial basis. In July of 1998, when Mr. Wang gave a speech in Japan, my family sent me the tape. After carefully listening to that tape, I bet my life on China No. 1 Tian Xian Liquid.

The doctor told me that when the cancer spread to the liver, I would not have lived any longer. My abdomen had been already filled with water. I thought, if I didn't go home then, I might not have another chance so I left the hospital. After one month of regularly using China No. 1 Tian Xian Liquid, the jaundice production and water accumulation in my abdomen began to recede. The drainage treatment wasn't necessary after the fourth month. Now a small bit of cancer tumor remains in my body but the bile duct inflammation and liver functions are getting better. This experience is beyond my wildest dreams.

Triumph Over Intestinal Cancer

Niece announces the amazing effect of China No. 1 Tian Xian Liquid
Kawada Takayuki (Aged 61, Hiroshima City, Hiroshima, Japan)

In February of 1995, the blood in my stool alarmed me and my family urged me to have an examination at hospital. The results showed that it was a rectum cancer and immediate surgery was necessary. Fortunately, the surgery became successful and I went home after a month.

I kept using the medication after hospitalization, even if I had to suffer from the side effects. Six months later, my niece who had suffered from cervical cancer told me that China No. 1 Tian Xian Liquid had cured her! So I began to use it. After six months, I was cured.

It has been four years now and I have examinations twice a year. None of them has shown any sign of abnormality. My life is back to normal.

When I visited Hong Kong with my wife in May 1998, I went to the global agent China-Japan Feida Union Co., Ltd. and asked all kinds of questions about the formula and I am very secured now using China No. 1 Tian Xian Liquid.

I use China No. 1 Tian Xian Liquid everyday, and my condition is getting better and better. Physically, I'm better than ever before. After I was cured, I traveled all around and I don't feel tired anymore. The joy of regaining health is unexplainable.

Now, I decreased the dosage but I still use it everyday and think of it as a healthcare supplement.

Triumph Over Intestinal Cancer

Easily Absorbed in the Human Body and the Effect is Amazing

Zhang Geng Min (Aged 75, Zhengzhou, Honen, China)

In Autumn of 1996, my stool became progressively smaller. I had a very uncomfortable bowel movement which was extremely painful. The condition worsened in February and I discovered blood in my stool. I went to the hospital for an examination.

After various examinations, the doctor told me it was ulcerous rectum cancer. I underwent radiotherapy and chemotherapy for two months. I went home when signs and symptoms stopped.

However, the rectum cancer recurred in 1998 and an endoscopy examination showed that the tumor had grown. It was confirmed by the CEA 7 mg/ml. However, I was too old for a surgery.

My family was very worried so they brought me China No.1 Tian Xian Liquid, China No. 1 Tian Xian Capsule and China No. 1 Tian Xian Suppository. It was recommended by an herbal doctor. I began to use them and in about three months, my bowel movement became smooth and the blood in my stool disappeared. A CT scan taken last January showed that the tumor was gone and CEA turned negative.

I continue to use China No. 1 Tian Xian Liquid and China No. 1 Tian Xian Suppository. It has been three years now since I was diagnosed of cancer and there are no signs of recurrence. China No. 1 Tian Xian Liquid is my savior, I am healthier than ever before. Having complete energy is the best of all feelings.

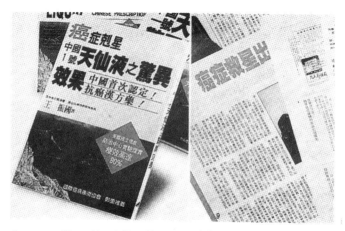

Learning China No. 1 Tian Xian Liquid from magazines, Mrs. Chen recommends it to Mr. Chen.

Triumph Over Intestinal Cancer

For the Sake of My Family, Never Surrender to Cancer
Fred Walter (Aged 52, truck driver, L.A., USA)

My CONDITION was getting worse when I lost weight and couldn't drive. An examination at the LA Public Hospital showed that I might have cancer. They arranged for me to undergo a CT scan at a cancer specialty hospital and their diagnosis confirmed that it was intestinal cancer. Man is a strange animal. I felt severe abdominal pain on the day when the diagnosis came out. It was a terminal cancer and surgery was immediately necessary. My Chinese mother-in-law knows that China No. 1 Tian Xian Liquid was a famous anti cancer Chinese medicine and she sent me some. The surgery took place on April 5, 1998.

Chemotherapy immediately followed the surgery and I began to use China No. 1 Tian Xian Liquid at the same time. Although the surgery had removed most part of the affected tissues, cancer cells remained in the lymph gland with the possibility to recur. The doctor told me about all the side effects of radiotherapy and chemotherapy and I was very lucky not to experience them.

I continue to use China No. 1 Tian Xian Liquid after the surgery and the cancer cells which remained in my body were removed. To date, there was a recurrence. I lost a great deal of weight during the ordeal. During the first six months after surgery, I regained my lost weight from 50kg to 70kg. Now, I feel more energetic than ever before.

We are eight in the family (my wife, four children and parents) I need to continue working for the next five or ten years before I retire. To prevent the recurrence of cancer, I use China No. 1 Tian Xian Liquid everyday.

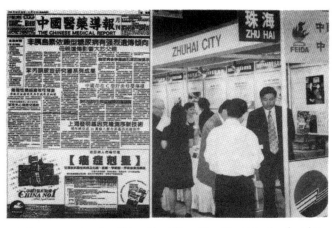

Information related to China No. 1 Tian Xian Liquid is also found in Chinese newspapers in the USA.

TRIUMPH OVER INTESTINAL CANCER

THANKS TO CHINA NO. 1 TIAN XIAN LIQUID, NORMAL
FAMILY LIFE RESUMES
Rick Mabin (Aged 62, Operations Consultant,
New York, USA)

BEFORE MY forties, I suffered from diabetes. After trying all kinds of medication, my life went bad. My doctor advised me to have further examinations but I left that because my diabetes doctor said that these conditions are quite normal for patients with diabetes.

In June of 1992, the condition worsened and I was referred to another hospital where I was diagnosed with hepatitis C. I was hospitalized immediately and they gave me anti-hepatitis vaccine everyday. The high

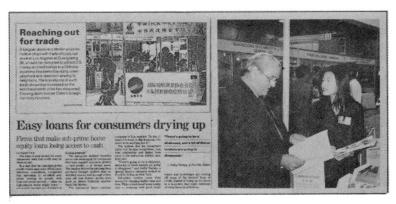

Information related to Exhibits of China No. 1 Tian Xian products are also published in American newspapers.

fever in the beginning was really annoying but I attributed it to the medicines. I did not stay long in the hospital. When we returned home from a family trip in the following year, I found blood in my stool one morning. An examination concluded that it was intestinal cancer. Surgery and hospitalization followed. They removed about 1.5 cm of my intestine and the doctor said that it was a pity that I did not discover it earlier.

I went back to work for about a year but I was so tired that I could only lie down resting most of the time. It was not long I was hospitalized for liver cancer. Both chemotherapy and surgery were administered. I had a ten-hour surgery and the doctor told me that the intestinal cancer had spread.

I suffered a lot from the accumulation of water in the abdomen during the surgery. In April, I chanced upon learning about the amazing China No. 1 Tian Xian Liquid from a news story. My daughter ordered some from Hong Kong immediately. On April 16, they used a urination medicine to discharge the water in my abdomen which resulted in discharging 2000ml on April 19. As a result, protein is lost but they used some kind of special machine to supplement protein through dripping. My insurance did not cover all the costs and I had to pay US$2,000.00 for each treatment.

The lymph duct was possibly infected and another probing surgery was necessary. Although nothing was found in the lymph duct, the surgery confirmed the cancer had spread to the liver. I did not have much time to live.

I increased the dosage of China No. 1 Tian Xian Liquid to six bottles a day and few days later, unusual white substances came out from the tubes connected to my body.

My doctor told me that I could go home if I want to. This was frightening to hear I thought this meant that I was going to die soon. I don't think he knew what the substance was. Maybe it was a product of the China No. 1 Tian Xian Liquid. The water in my abdomen began to disappear and related procedures to extract them was suspended. About a month later, all the tubes used to discharge the fluid were removed and I went home in February.

Then I regained my energy and my normal life resumed. Thank you, China No. 1 Tian Xian Liquid.

TRIUMPH OVER INTESTINAL CANCER

SURPRISING EFFECTS FOUND DURING EARLY STAGE OF CANCER

Lin Su Feng (Aged 54, High School teacher, Tainan, Taiwan)

I SUFFERED from severe diarrhea in February 1998 and lost 8 kg for no apparent reason. I went to the Chengkung University Hospital for an examination of a bleeding anus and I was diagnosed with intestinal cancer.

According to the doctors, blood stool was a typical symptom for intestinal cancer. Many people have mistaken it as sign of hemorrhoids and therefore cannot detect cancer in its early stage.

Immediate hospitalization and surgery were arranged and my co-workers recommended China No. 1 Tian Xian Liquid before the surgery.

In fact, they told me that a friend's wife recovered from breast cancer by using it. So I accepted their recommendation without any doubt.

Details about China No. 1 Tian Xian Liquid were obtained from Hong Kong global agent and it included successful case histories from around the world. I hoped that it can cure me, too.

Radiotherapy and chemotherapy were administered and at the same time China No. 1 Tian Xian Liquid and China No. 1 Tian Xian Capsule were used at the same time. Six months later, after an examinatio, everything returned to normal and I am still using China No. 1 Tian Xian Liquid and China No. 1 Tian Xian Capsule.

By using them, side effects of the radiotherapy and chemotherapy were greatly reduced and I recovered faster and better than other patients with similar condition.

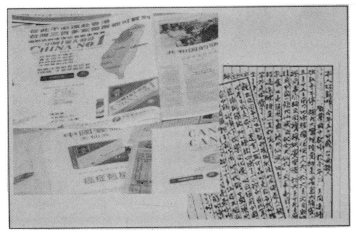

Testimonials and doctor's reports from Hong Kong and Taiwan clients.

Triumph Over Esophagus Cancer

Tumor with diameter of 10cm almost
disappears
Ting Su Ying (aged 70, HK)

I RETIRED fifteen years ago and I just stayed home to take care of my grandchildren and enjoy the rest of my life. I felt there was something wrong with my throat three years ago when I vomited and a bad feeling emerged.

I did not take heed at first but a swallowing problem gradually worsened. My daughter accompanied me for an examination and the X-ray showed that there was a 10-cm tumor in the middle of my esophagus. The doctor told me that I was too old for surgery so I underwent radiotherapy and chemotherapy. In spite of the therapies, the swallowing problem persisted aside from the side effects of the therapies. I felt it was the end of my life.

At that time, my son-in-law learned of the anti cancer effect of China No.1 Tian Xian Liquid so he bought me some.

After two weeks of using China No. 1 Tian Xian Liquid, I could take in liquid food. After about a month, all the side effects were gone and I was able to eat soft food. Three months later, an X-ray examination showed that the tumor reduced in size by one third. The doctor was surprised and claimed that it was due to the effect of the therapies. However, I firmly believe that it was the work of China No. 1 Tian Xian Liquid.

It's been three years now, I am fully recovered.

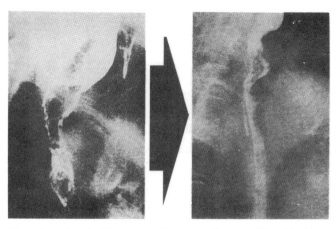

X-ray shows that the 10-cm tumor disappears after using China No. 1 Tian Xian Liquid.

TRIUMPH OVER ESOPHAGUS CANCER

ESOPHAGUS CANCER IS CURED WHEN
OPERATION IS IMPOSSIBLE
Ma Guan Ren (Aged 53, Service industry, Nanyang City, Henan, China)

IT STARTED as uneasiness while eating. The condition persisted for about two months and swallowing became increasingly difficult. On October 23, 1996, I'll never forget, when I was diagnosed with esophagus cancer. I was immediately hospitalized at the Henan Tumor Hospital for treatment of a 5.5 cm tumor. The doctors said that surgery was impossible.

After two months of chemotherapy and radiotherapy, there were no signs of recovery. The barium milk test in March 1997 confirmed that the tumor had grown to 8.5 cm big.

I was anxious about the therapies and when I learned about China No. 1 Tian Xian Liquid from the news, I tried it. In less than two weeks, the swallowing problem had greatly improved, chest pain was relieved, and my over all condition got better. I left the hospital on March 27.

I kept on using China No. 1 Tian Xian Liquid after I went home. The swallowing problems disappeared, the chest pain gone, and all other symptoms faded. I followed the dietary instructions given by Mr. Wang and I regained my appetite and gradually gained back 15kg. A barium milk test in July showed that everything was normal. In November of 1998 an examination confirmed that there was no sign of recurrence.

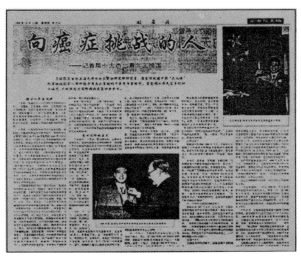

News coverage about the effects of China No. 1 Tian Xian Liquid on esophagus cancer

TRIUMPH OVER LIVER CANCER

NEVER SURRENDER EVEN WHEN OPERATIONS FAIL
Nishimura Zentaro (Aged 83, Kyoto, Japan)

MY LIVER cancer was discovered during a check up at the Central Hospital in November of 1992. I was hospitalized at the National Cancer Center in December and their examination showed that I am also suffering from stomach cancer. The doctor told me that surgery would be very difficult because the cancer was located in two separate organs and I was too old to withstand it. Even if I insisted on having surgery, I would only have few months to live.

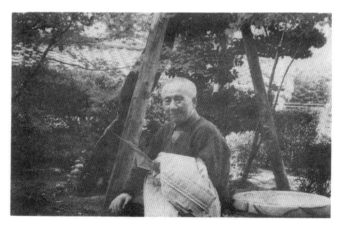

"It is a surprise to live with cancer in peace," exclaimed the doctor.

However, I did not feel uncomfortable at that time and I was not depressed. I could not stand the diarrhea brought about by the medications. After talking with the doctor, I stopped all the medications. I started looking for alternative medicines or prescriptions that may cure my disease. After learning of China No. 1 Tian Xian Liquid from my daughter, I bought some through my friend in Hong Kong.

It has been six years now and I've never stopped using it. The monthly examinations, including checks on liver, kidney, white blood cells, and hemoglobin are all normal. My worry about stomach cancer is gone and all the pain is gone. My friend teases me and calls me "superman." Even the doctor exclaims that, "it is a surprise to live with cancer whithout pain."

Six years ago, I was told that I had only a few months to live and toay there was nothing abnormal today. I will never forget the grace that China No. 1 Tian Xian Liquid has brought. I don't know how long I will live but with China No. 1 Tian Xian Liquid, I will never surrender.

Triumph Over Liver Cancer

In just a blink of the eye you will be more ener-
getic than other normal people
Igeta Toshikazv (Aged 51, Office clerk, Kitaadachi, Saitama,
Japan/reported by his wife)

My husband had a liver problem and needed to receive regular treatment. One day, his condition got worse and I suggested that he be examined at a hospital. The result showed that it was a terminal cancer and we were told that he will have only two to three months to live. I could not believe it, I was in a state of shock.

He came home two months later with loss of confidence and emotionally drained. The family was trying to maintain a normal life by being very cautious not to cause him any unnecessary stress. No matter what happens, we would tolerate him because we wanted to be with him.

My husband knew that I began looking for anything that could cure him. He learned about China No. 1 Tian Xian Liquid and he bought some immediately.

To my surprise, he got much better after using it for a short time. He is now better than ever before. Now he works harder than ever before for his beloved family.

Whenever our family or friends have medical problems, we will recommend China No. 1 Tian Xian Liquid. Although the tumor is still there, it has become very small.

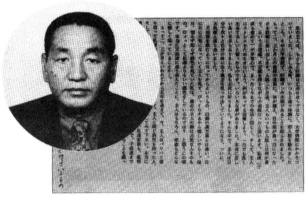

Igeta in desperate search of a cure for his liver cancer.

Triumph Over Liver Cancer

Recurrence of Cancer After Reducing the Dosage
Dota Isamu (Aged 69, Itabash, Tokyo)

IT WAS ten years ago when my liver problem turned out to be cancer. The size of the tumor was 1 x 2cm. I went to the hospital very often to receive all kinds of treatment, including ethanol injections. None of them worked.

After two or three years, I learned about China No. 1 Tian Xian Liquid from the magazines. After collecting more information about it, I decided to use it. The result was immediate. The ultrasound examination in October of 1993 showed the shadow had disappeared. Then I reduced the dosage to two bottles a day.

In another examination of October 1997, the tumor reappeared to a size at 1.2cm. Then I resumed the original dosage and in an examination of October 1998, there was no sign of the tumor and everything returned to normal.

CONTINUE USING CHINA NO. 1 TIAN XIAN LIQUID TO PREVENT RECURRENCE.

Namiki Hide (Aged 78, Hiroshima City, Hiroshima, Japan/ reported by the husband)

IN NOVEMBER of 1995, she went for an ultrasound examination which showed a shadow of tumor. A CT scan in January, the doctor found a 4 x 4cm liver tumor. She went to the hospital to receive the suppository treatment because she was too old to undergo surgery.

However, none of the treatments worked and she was discharged in April. We learned of China No. 1 Tian Xian Liquid from a news story and we immediately bought some.

After a week's hospitalization in June, China No. 1 Tian Xian Liquid arrived. At the same time when the suppository treatment was administered, she began using the liquid. She was fully recovered in two weeks time. A month later, an examination showed that the tumor had reduced in size. Doctors then advised her to use the suppository treatment continuously but we rejected it because of her old age. We did however, continue to give her China No. 1 Tian Xian Liquid. In January of 1996, an examination showed the tumor had disappeared.

In fact, we stopped giving her China No. 1 Tian Xian Liquid

for almost two years after her recovery but later recurred. Now, we're using the suppository treatment and China No. 1 Tian Xian Liquid. The liver cancer recurred very easily so I still give her two bottles a day. We believe that the success in her case is the result of China No. 1 Tian Xian Liquid.

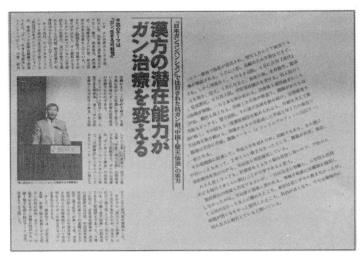

I learn about China No. 1 Tian Xian Liquid from the media.

Triumph Over Liver Cancer

It accelerates stability during the post-operation healing
Yokokawa Kenki (Aged 67, Hiratsuka, Kanagawa, Japan)

I was not healthy and I needed a lot of rest very often. I always had colds and suffer from constipation.

In summer of 1994, I was diagnosed with hepatitis C after an examination. The diagnosis was changed to cirrhosis. I received a spleen removal surgery the following year and doctors discovered a tumor in my liver. They gave me an ethanol injection.

The condition got worse and the tumor expanded. They removed one third of my liver and the gall bladder. In 1997, they changed the diagnosis to multiple liver cancer after I had received five surgeries. I began using China No. 1 Tian Xian Liquid after the second surgery. Thanks to it, I recovered from the surgeries very fast. I regained my appetite, and more importantly, it hindered the growth of the tumor.

Triumph Over Liver Cancer

Continuous spreading of liver cancer recovered
Gondo Masako (Aged 51, Hyogo, Japan)

I RECEIVED a breast cancer surgery twelve years ago. Three years later, it spread to my ovary, which was removed during the second surgery. Cancer cells were still inside my body. My lung was infected three years later. Had I not been advised by my doctor to undergo immediate surgery, the cancer cells would have spread throughout the entire body. I decided to have the third surgery.

I had a follow up chemotherapy once a week but it didn't work. I lost my confidence and appetite. They discovered a new tumor (3cm.) in my body during a CT scan.

The doctor said there was little hope. After consulting with the doctors about Chinese medicine, we received a suggestion to use China No. 1 Tian Xian Liquid. I had no knowledge of Chinese medicine at that time. It was my family who encouraged me to try it.

I remembered the first time I used it on November 16, 1997. In just two weeks, I regained my energy and appetite.

In the beginning of 1998, I took 20ml twice a day and I had weekly examination. By October, the 3 cm tumor reduced to 1 cm and my blood was normal. This case has amazed the doctors.

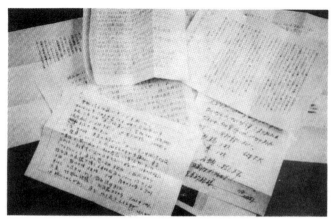

Overcoming liver cancer by using China No. 1 Tian Xian Liquid

TRIUMPH OVER LIVER CANCER

NO MORE THAN SIX MONTHS TO LIVE, CHINA NO. 1 TIAN XIAN LIQUID IS THE LAST HOPE.
Cheng Chi Keung (Aged 67, HK)

IT HAPPENED about a year ago when I started itching all over my whole body. I went to the hospital and they told my wife about the result of the examination. She looked very strange and reluctantly told me the truth at my instance.

It was a liver cancer. The doctor said that I had no more than six months to live. Radiation therapy or chemotherapy may extend my life for another two years if everything went right.

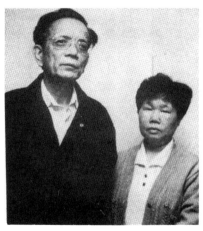

Mr. & Mrs. Cheng told their story.

I was stunned upon hearing this and I was in complete denial. I received both therapies to live longer but they only added to my suffering.

I was lucky to learn about China No. 1 Tian Xian Liquid from my friends. My wife and daughter told me not to worry about money. They just wanted me to try anything that may help. I began using it because I did not want to let them down. Somehow, something unbelievable happened to me. I was getting better.

I regained my appetite. The irritation and itching disappeared. I could sleep throughout the night.

I stopped using Western medicine altogether replacing it with the China No. 1 Tian Xian Liquid everyday. I decided to beat cancer. As long as one has the energy, there is hope to overcome cancer. Even though the itching is still there still I feel energetic and healthy.

Triumph Over Liver Cancer

Recovered from Useless Operation
Kong Tie Guan (Aged 47, Functionary,
Shanghai, China)

I FELT abdominal pain and pressure and I lost a great deal of weight due to jaundice.

I had an examination on April 22, 1998. The findings concluded that I had a liver cancer and a surgery followed immediately. Everything went satisfactorily and I went home very soon. I had fever and pain for a month so I went back to the hospital. After series of examinations; an ultrasound, a CT scan, tumor probes, alpha fetoproteins (AFP) analysis and liver function tests, they confirmed the recurrence of my liver cancer.

It is very difficult to detect changes in liver cancer and when it was discovered, it is often to late for surgery. I am the best example. Because I wanted to spend my last days with my family. I went home without any therapy. The condition got worse during this period.

I then went to Mr. Wang's clinic and he immediately gave me a three month prescription of China No. 1 Tian Xian Liquid. The fever decreased, energy level increased and my appetite has resumed. A further examination showed that the tumor got smaller and everything was normal.

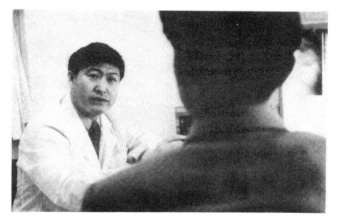

Mr. Kong decided to use China No. 1 Tian Xian Liquid after the diagnosis by Mr. Wang.

Triumph Over Liver Cancer

True Feelings of Being Cured Right After Using
China No. 1 Tian Xian Liquid
Tang Yi Chen (Aged 54, Functionary, Guangdong)

In September of 1997, my abdominal pain began. I lost my appetite and I experienced severe pain in the morning of November 29.

A CT scan confirmed a liver cancer and a 1.5 x 6 cm tumor. I already lost 20kgs.

I couldn't survive for two more months and there wasn't any cancer specialist in the hospital. Neither radiotherapy nor chemotherapy was available.

Later my family heard about Mr. Wang in Zhuhai City. They visited his clinic and bought some China No. 1 Tian Xian Liquid, China No. 1 Tian Xian Capsule and China No. 1 Tian Xian Suppository. I took 10ml of the liquid three times a day, five capsules three times a day, and one suppository twice a day.

In about a week's time, the severe abdominal pain began to recede. In December, a CT scan showed that the tumor had shrunk to 3 x 4 cm. I felt much better than before.

I visited Mr. Wang again and he advised me to use maximum dosage of China No. 1 Tian Xian Liquid.

In February of 1998, I could feel that my condition was improving. On April 10, the CT scan showed that the tumor had reduced to 2 x 2cm. All other symptoms were gone.

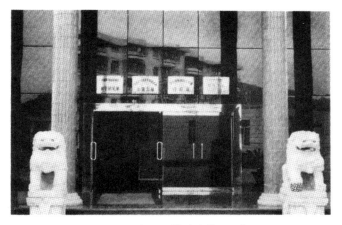

Mr. Wang's clinic in Zhuhai, Guangzhou

Triumph Over Liver Cancer

How Lucky I am to Know Dr. Wang and China No. 1 Tian Xian Liquid
Dong Hai Ben (Aged 54, Service industry. Qian An, Jilin, China)

There was a fist-size lump on the right hand side of my abdomen. It was painful especially whenever touched. I felt very tired. I lost my appetite and painful constipation and diarrhea kept on recurring. I lost almost all my energy.

There is no tumor specialty hospital in Jilin but we have Mr. Wang of Jilin, his hometown. I went to his Institute in August of 1996 and they confirmed the presence of a 14 x 9cm. tumor in my liver.

Mr. Wang asked me why I waited so long to ask for help as my condition was getting critical. I could die at any moment. I must thank Mr. Wang for telling me the seriousness of my situation.

I began using China No. 1 Tian Xian Liquid. Fifty days later, the condition greatly improved. The tumor got smaller and I could a walk and do some light work.

I knew that I was about to die but using China No. 1 Tian Xian Liquid has cured me. In February of 1997, a CT scan showed that there was nothing abnormal. A year later, liver pain disappeared. I completely recovered and everything returned to normal.

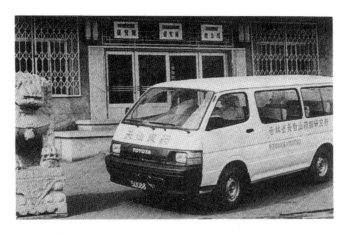

Changbai Mountain Pharmacology Research Institute and Clinic in Tonghua, Jilin.

TRIUMPH OVER LIVER CANCER

THANKS GOD FOR LETTING ME REALIZE THE BEAUTY OF LIFE
Hun Yuan (Aged 58, Writer, Taipei, Taiwan)

I SUFFERED from cancer disease three times for the last twelve years. First, it was breast cancer, then cervical cancer and finally liver cancer. The fear of physical pain and dying made me realize how vulnerable I am.

When I look back at my struggles against cancer, I feel like a grass standing in the midst of strong winds and I grow in the warmth of the sun. Life is now more important and more beautiful than before.

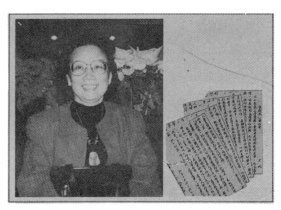

"Life is so important to me", said Jun Yuan.

Modern medicine did little to control my disease! The side effects of the therapies made me suffer more than the disease itself. Sometimes I want to give up and die. Thanks to a great medical team that encouraged and helped me through the darkest moment of my life. I have survived and now I feel that life has more meaning.

My father and his herbal doctor friend told me about the effectiveness of combining Chinese and Western medicines in cancer treatment. So I used Chinese medicine to relieve the side effects of the Western medicine. It was the source of hope. I began to use China No. 1 Tian Xian Liquid.

It helped to relieve all the side effects and improved my energy levels. Both the doctor and my friends were astonished how I overcome cancer. Now to live life is not my only goal. I want to help all other patients by giving them courage.

TRIUMPH OVER LUNG CANCER

FOREVER GRATITUDE TO CHINA NO. 1 TIAN XIAN LIQUID
RECOMMENDED BY MY FRIEND STAYING IN THE SAME HOSPITAL.
Watanabe Yuki (Aged 58, Housewife, Hashiki, Japan)

I BEGAN coughing severely in November of 1997 and I thought it was flu. I went to the hospital and they gave me some anti-cough medicine. Coughing did not stop after two weeks.

I had an X-ray examination at another hospital and it showed the accumulation of liquid in my lungs. It was the cause of my cough. They drained 4.5 liters of the water in the hospital.

The severe cough recurred in April of 1998 and water accumulation in my lungs was again confirmed. After draining the water in the left lung, I thought I could go home. But water began to accumulate in the right lung as well. I had another operation and they injected my lungs with medication to prevent further water accumulation.

However, my body rejected the medication and I suffered from high fever and difficulty in breathing. I was roaming around the entrance of hell for three days. The treatment for the right lung was suspended and the cough wouldn't go away. I lost all my appetite.

The cough became increasingly worst after I went home. It was even difficult for me to climb the stairs.

I suffered greatly from the severe cough during the three weeks of stay at home. Then I went back to the hospital again. On July 15, the final test results confirmed of my lung cancer.

The severe cough made it difficult for me to speak, breathe, and walk so I was bedridden. At that time, the patient next to me told me about China No. 1 Tian Xian Liquid.

I began taking four bottles a day. In just three days, the severe cough was slightly relieved. I even had enough strength to walk to the toilet.

On September 13, I thought I would be able to attend my daughter's wedding. However, I felt I was recovering and I thought that maybe China No. 1 Tian Xian Liquid would have made it possible. On July 23, they gave me anti cancer drip treatment many people had warned me about the severe side effects of such treatment.

My dream came true, I managed to attend the wedding from the hospital. I left the hospital on October 15 and follow-up x-ray examination showed that lung cancer had disappeared and without any water accumulation. My friend and I will always thank China No. 1 Tian Xian Liquid.

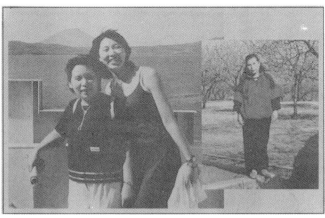

*I must recover to join the **wedding** of my daughter ...! the brave Mrs. Watanabe and her daughter.*

Triumph Over Lung Cancer

Return to work right after recovery
Yamada Kimihiko (aged 41, Chiba,
Japan/reported by his wife)

In November of 1983, my husband received surgery for thyroid cancer. In 1992, it was confirmed that the cancer had spread to his lungs, brain and neck. Surgery followed. As cancer cells had already expanded to both lungs, surgery was impossible. The doctor told me that he would only live for another three to four years.

About three years ago, a friend advised him to try dietary treatment. I stopped it because I thought it would cause other problems. However, I did not restrict his diet since he was afflected with lung cancer in 1995, he regained back his energy. During the same winter, he lost his voice. In February of 1996, he had bloody phlegm in an isotope examination.

He was then hospitalized. I kept thinking 'what else can we do.' I then remembered something about China No. 1 Tian Xian Liquid so I looked into the details. After confirming the 80% curative rate I pin all my hope on it. I ordered some from Hong Kong.

My husband had no faith in it and he refused to try any Chinese medicine because we already had a lot of them. China No. 1 Tian Xian Liquid was delivered to our home five days after we placed the order. It was my last hope so I encouraged him to try. He used eight bottles a day when he was hospitalized and his condition began to improve so we left the hospital. He continued using it. Ten days later, the bloody phlegm stopped, chest pain disappeared in another week and regained both his voice and his energy. He went back to work immediately although the cancer is still there, his condition is very stable.

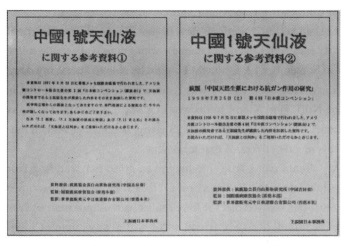

Information about China No. 1 Tian Xian Liquid from Mr. Wang's office in Japan.

Triumph Over Lung Cancer

Three Years Ago, I Was Told to Have No Less Than A Year to Live
Ishikawa Hideko (Aged 67, Housewife, Kyoto, Japan/
reported by her husband)

In July of 1997, my wife was diagnosed of lung cancer and surgery was confirmed impossible. They gave her chemotherapy and radiotherapy. The doctor suspected that she has less than a year to live.

After undergoing chemotherapy in October, my wife became very weak from the side effects. She could not stand it. Approximately 20% of the cancer cells was still there. In late October, radiotherapy was resumed when there were signs of recurrence in late October. The therapy continued throughout December and cancer was still there. As there was no sign of pain, she went home in late December.

Then May of 1998, an examination showed that cancer cells had already spread to her brain. She was hospitalized immediately to receive chemotherapy and radiotherapy. The cancer was still in her lung and brain. The therapy has ended in late June. In consideration of my wife's physical condition, the doctor told us that no more therapy should be given. In other words, it was a hopeless case.

We learned about China No. 1 Tian Xian Liquid from the news and I immediately bought some. My wife has suffered from gastritis which resulted from building pressure, I gave her two bottles a day starting in late May. I changed it to four bottles a day in June and her stomach pain receded. In July, the examination showed that her lung cancer was still present but the cancer in the brain had disappeared.

Frankly speaking, China No. 1 Tian Xian Liquid was not the only medication we have ever tried. For my wife, I have tried almost everything but the result was in vain. We learned about China No. 1 Tian Xian Liquid when she was hospitalized.

China No. 1 Tian Xian Liquid is really amazing. It can cure cancer that cannot be cured by Western therapy. After we have tried everything, we discovered that it was very effective. In just a month or so, her brain cancer disappeared much to our great surprise. Thanks to China No. 1 Tian Xian Liquid.

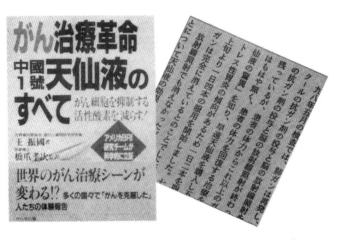

Books and mail talking about China No. 1 Tian Xian Liquid.

Although the brain cancer had gone, the lung cancer was still there. To avoid its progression, we continue to use China No. 1 Tian Xian Liquid.

To improve energy, we've also used China No. 1 Tian Xian Capsule No. 3 since August. She left the hospital in mid August and we took the doctor's advice to use stomach medication in combination with China No. 1 Tian Xian products.

Because of China No. 1 Tian Xian Liquid, my wife is still alive.

TRIUMPH OVER LUNG CANCER

NO SIGN OF RECURRENCE AFTER THE OPERATION FIVE YEARS AGO
Jian Yong Guang (Aged 70, Deputy Director, National Defense Ministry, ROC)

AFTER A regular check up in April of 1995, I was diagnosed with stage two of lung cancer. Immediate surgery was necessary I would only survive in less than five years. It was so sudden that no one could accept it. I jogged 10km a day to keep healthy and I had regular check ups because I am a retired military officer.

I was a soldier and death does not frighten me but when I learned about it I kept asking, 'why me?' There were no symptoms at all.

I was hospitalized and operated in May. Although they removed part of my left lung, the surgery did not completely remove the cancer.

The doctor then advised me to undergo chemotherapy to prevent it from spreading. I refused, but I am not afraid of death, I am a man of strength. I was not afraid of the pains of the therapy I just wanted to wait for sometime.

I turned down chemotherapy. I could not go out in this manner. I could accept death but I would never surrender.

After surgery, my condition became extremely worse. The wounds hurt badly and even lumped. Of course, I lost my energy, appetite, and weight.

Then I heard that my friend's wife was cured by a Chinese medicine so I looked into it. She explained the details of China No. 1 Tian Xian Liquid to me and because of her acquaintance with Mr. Wang, she could inquire from him about my condition.

The encouragement came from Mr. Wang, "don't feel hopeless, you can always be cured!' He also sent me instructions how to use China No. 1 Tian Xian Liquid and I began taking it immediately. I witnessed the miracle on my friend's wife so I believe I have hope, too. The pain was gone away after using it in just a short time but I began itching and had diarrhea for 2 months. To tell you the truth, I was not sure if I recovered or not. According to Mr. Wang, it was normal and I trusted him.

In an examination seven months after, the surgery showed that the cancer cells had disappeared and everything was normal. I still use China No. 1 Tian Xian Liquid and I enjoy a happy and healthy life.

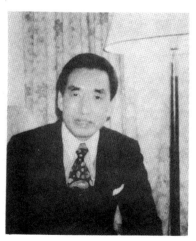

Mr. Jiang no recurrence after the surgery 5 years ago.

TRIUMPH OVER LUNG CANCER

I REGAINED MY LIFE THROUGH THE INFORMATION NETWORK
Liu Wai (Aged 55, guard, HK)

I AM a physically fit person and I could not believe that I am suffering from cancer. I went to the hospital for further examination for chronic cough in September of 1996. Lung cancer was confirmed and surgery followed despite my refusal.

I knew nothing about my condition not until after four months. They gave me radiotherapy and chemotherapy. I lost almost all my hair. The doctor continued the therapies.

About the same time, my son learned about China No. 1 Tian Xian

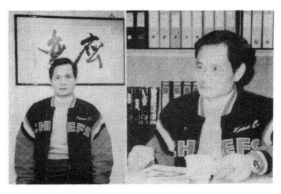

Mr. Lau says, "the combined use of Western medicine and China No. 1 Tian Xian Liquid is amazing!"

Liquid from the Internet. I bought some. I don't discriminate against Chinese Medicine but since the doctors do not recognize it, I used it secretly.

It was costly to have both therapies at the same time so I asked the doctor to stop the chemotherapy.

I began using China No. 1 Tian Xian Liquid. My condition was getting better and my hair began to grow again. I told my doctor about this when I stopped coughing but he had already suspected it. It was difficult for him to believe it. The miracle came from the combination of China No. 1 Tian Xian Liquid, chemotherapy and radiotherapy.

I began using China No. 1 Tian Xian suppository in June of 1998 with dramatic effects. The lung cancer receded and I went back to work. My overall condition was getting better.

However, pain was still there after the surgery so I also used China No. 1 Tian Xian Plaster to relieve the pain. I must take care of my family. I have to work. That was my reasoning and motivation to get cured.

The doctor said that the tumor condition was stable and I only needed to have an examination once a month. The chemotherapy was stopped. To maintain my weight and health, I went to China Japan Feida Union Co., Ltd. (the global agent of China No. 1 Tian Xian Liquid) to ask for dietary treatment instruction. As long as it helps, I'll try everything.

I am the only survivor among all cancer patients receiving care from the hospital when I was there. Thanks to China No. 1 Tian Xian Liquid, I am still alive. The Chinese should not discriminate against Chinese medicine. When used in conjunction with Western medicine, it can improve the survival rate.

I started smoking at the age of ten and lung cancer became unavoidable. I have changed now. I quit smoking and I advise you not to smoke.

178

Triumph Over Lung Cancer

Just After a Year of Using China No. 1 Tian Xian Liquid, the Tumor Completely Disappeared.

Zhu Yu Lan (Aged 49, service industry, Siping, Jilin, China)

A fever, a cough, bloody phlegm and chest pain began on December 3, 1995. An x-ray examination showed there was a 3 x 4 cm tumor in my left lung and cancer cells were also found in my phlegm.

I received radiotherapy at the hospital. It was not effective. I left the hospital on the 8th of February 1996. I was very anxious.

In July of 1996, a friend of mine overcame stomach cancer with China No. 1 Tian Xian Liquid. After she told me about her recovery. I began using it. In about two months, the symptoms were gone and the tumor had reduced to 2 x 3 cm.

I continued using it and in August of 1997, an x-ray examination showed the tumor was gone. The CEA was also negative. There was no sign of recurrence. With China No. 1 Tian Xian Liquid, I feel more energetic than ever.

TRIUMPH OVER LUNG CANCER

IN LESS THAN FIVE MONTHS, THE TUMOR DISAPPEARED
AND I AM BACK TO NORMAL.
Wang Zhou Hong (Aged 63, shop owner, Malaysia)

IN MARCH of 1997, I had an x-ray examination and further examinations revealed that I am suffering from lung cancer. They found a benign 3 x 2 cm tumor. The decision on surgery depended on the results of the examinations. Surgery is never good for the elderly so I took medication treatment instead..

In May, my son learned from the Internet that Mr. Wang was coming to Malaysia to give free consultation, so I went to see him. Mr. Wang immediately confirmed the lung cancer diagnosis and prescribed a one month treatment program of China No. 1 Tian Xian Liquid, China No. 1 Tian Xian Capsule, and China No. 1 Tian Xian Plaster. In June, an examination showed that the tumor reduced to half of the original size. The effect was amazing.

Then in October 25, x-ray examination showed that it was completely gone. My joy was ineffable. It was China No. 1 Tian Xian Liquid that protected me from the horrors of pain.

Although the tumor is gone, I still use China No. 1 Tian Xian Liquid to prevent any recurrence. An examination in March of 1998, reconfirmed that everything is normal. I became increasingly better.

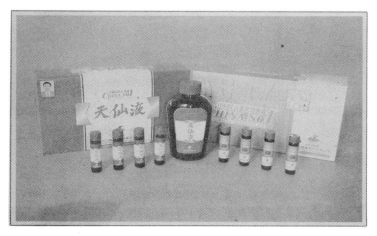

China No. 1 Tian Xian Liquid and its sister product - Natural Nutritions Liquid

Triumph Over Lung Cancer

Shadows in the lung vanished in two months.
Sing Kio (aged 67, merchant, Manila, Philippines)
April 23, 1998 - Century Park Sheraton Hotel, Manila,
Philippines

Good day to everyone. Today, I am here to share on how the Tian Xian Liquid has cured my cancer. First things first, I would like to make it known that I do not have any relation with Professor Wang Zhen Guo nor with Mr. Manuel Kiok (General Manager of Green & Gold International Exports).

I would also like to say that it is not Professor Wang nor Mr. Kiok who asked me to share my case. In fact, I volunteered. My primary motive in testifying here today is to listen to the lecture of Wang Zhen Guo on cancer. Secondly, I wish to personally thank Professor Wang Zhen Guo for his invention (China No. 1 New Tian Xian Liquid) which has cured my cancer disease.

Let me tell you how I was able to come to speak before you today. Sometime ago, I saw an advertisement of the Tian Xian Liquid and the Anti-Cancer Seminar (April 23, 1998) in a Chinese newspaper. I decided to call up the office of the distributor (Green & Gold International Exports). I was able to talk to Mr. Kiok personally. Eventually, I told him that I have been cured of cancer 7 years ago due to intake of the Tian Xian Liquid. I said I could share my testimony on the day of the lecture provided that my transportation will be made available.

Before I continue, I would like to testify that I wasn't able to undergo any surgery, chemotherapy, cobalt therapy or any other solution/medicine due to the position of the cancer (near my heart). I was left with no option but to depend on Chinese herbal medicine. (China No. 1 Tian Xian Liquid) Please see note below.

Last June 1991, there were nights while sleeping, I would cough very hard and throw up phlegm. Like normal procedure, I took common Western and Chinese herbal medicines to cure my simple disease.

But this did not solve the problem. I then consulted a physician named Dr. Ang. He's an old doctor and has a lot of experience. After taking an x-ray (Figure 1), the doctor noted a slight enlargement near my left lung. "This is a very suspicious area, you'll have to go get a CT-SCAN," the doctor suggested". I hesitated to have a CT-SCAN and I just asked the doctor to prescribe some medicine. He prescribed some antibiotics but unfortunately, it didn't work. I visited him again and he gave me another similar set of antibiotics only the names have been changed. But still, nothing has worked.

By November, I already had a fever. After realizing that the medicines have no effect, I went to see another doctor, coincidentally, his name is Dr. Ang. The second doctor was older than the first and was very popular during the 1950's. After showing my previous x-ray to the second doctor, he also gave me the same explanation and prescription. The medicine didn't work again. The second time I went back to the doctor, he prescribed me a new set of antibiotics. This time around, the medicine didn't conform with my body and hence, I lost 8 pounds.

I took the medicine from November 11 to December 10, 1981. But my fever worsened, my phlegm already contained blood, and my cough became worst. So I went out to look for another doctor in a big hospital. This time around, the doctor was a young one. On December 10, 1991, the third doctor advised me to have another x-ray and CT-SCAN. Two days later, I saw the result (Refer to Figure 2). The result was worse unimaginable. The doctor didn't even believe that the man who has the x-ray is still alive.

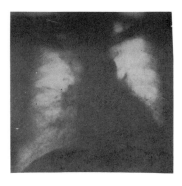

The tumor got worse. (December 10, 1991)

X-RAY CONSULTATION REPORT:

Chinese General Hospital and Medical Center.

Case No. 360114. Name: Sing Kio, Referred by: Dr. R. Ngo. Date: 12-10-91. Clinical Date: CHEST. Compared with the previous examination taken outside dated 11-11-91 shows interval progression of the atelectasis and infiltrates in the left lung base. The right lung is clear. Heart is not enlarged. Diaphragm is intact.

IMPRESSION: Atelectasis and pneumonia infiltrates, left lung base showing interval progression. Possibility of this being secondary to hilar compression cannot be ruled out.

By: E. Dy M.D. (Radiologist)

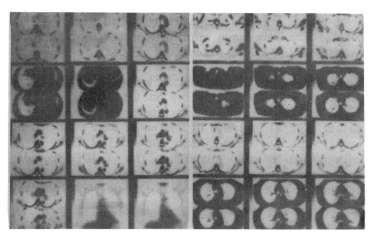

CT SCAN   CT-SCAN

CT-SCAN details: Chinese General Hospital & Medical Center, Section of computed Tomography. Name: Sing Kio. Age: 58. CT No.: 91-1870. Referred by: Dr. R. Ngo. Date: 12-20-91.

Consultation Report: C.T. SCAN OF THE CHEST. Contrast illustration of the chest shows a huge pulmonary mass in the left lower lobe measuring 9.4 x 6.4 cm. This is attached to the hilum and pleura. Nodular densities are seen in the he hilum. Acinar infiltrates are noted in the left upper lobe. Fibrotic densities are seen in both apices. The heart is lightly enlarged. No lytic changes demonstrated. IMPRESSION: Pulmonary mass, left lower lobe, malignancy is highly considered. Attachment to the hilum and pleura is demonstrated. Left hilar lymphadenopathy. Fibrosis, both apices.

By: Cesar S. Co. M.D.

At that time, someone has recommended the use of some basic Chinese medicine. Nothing changed in 20 days. Someone then recommended Tian Xian Liquid. After taking Tian Xian Liquid from January 10 till the end of February 1992 (approximately a month and a half), I had another x-ray (Refer to Figure 6). The doctor said that the results were much better than the previous ones (Refer to Figure 3) but still, this was a serious condition. My fever and cough have diminished and vanished eventually.

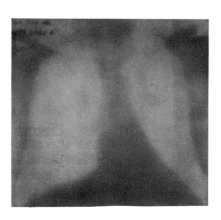

Result of my
continuous intake of
Tian Xian Liquid.
(June 29, 1992)

Analysis of X-RAY: Name: Sing Kio.
Age: 58. X-Ray No.: 5619. Date: 6-29-92.
Examination: *CHEST. Examination of the chest shows the heart to be normal in size. The aorta is slightly dilated. Blunting of the left costophrenic sulcus is noted. Apical pleural thickening is noted on the right. Minimal fibrosis is noted in both upper lung fields, more on the right. The finding appears to be inactive Koch's lesion. Comparison with previous study will be of help. Minimal fibrosis is also seen at the*

left base and could be due to residual change from previous pneumonia.

*   **Summary:** Examination of the chest shows minimal scar, both upper lung fields, appears to be inactive Koch's lesion. Minimal fibrosis at the left base is also noted.*

*   By: Lorna S. Yiu UP, M.D. Diplomate, American Board of Radiology and Nuclear Medicine. 645 Condesa Street, Binondo, Manila.*

Along with Tian Xian Liquid, I also eat fruits and drink vegetable juices (half slice carrots, apple, one third of a cucumber, long celery, 2-3 leaves of lettuce, sugar beet). After extracting the juices, I drank 3 glasses per day. I continued to take the Tian Xian Liquid until June of 1992 before I had another x-ray. My fever and cough have been cured. I took another x-ray (Figure 6) showed that there was nothing wrong with me. I took the x-ray on a commercial firm, not in the hospital. My tumor has vanished. The doctor said that it looked like a dry scar of tuberculosis. Then, I stopped taking the Tian Xian Liquid until now.

Last month (March 1998), I took another x-ray (Refer to Figure 7). The x-ray further confirmed that there is nothing wrong with me.

Recently I have been diagnosed with colon cancer. So in April 1998, I started taking up the Tian Xian Liquid again. The doctor advised me to undergo operation for my colon cancer. I refused and wanted to rely only on Tian Xian Liquid. I hope by next year, I could be here again and testify before you the wonders of Tian Xian Liquid. My contact number is with Mr. Manuel Kiok. Should you be interested to get any help or solicit any information, please don't hesitate to contact me.

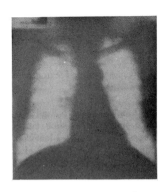

No Problem!
(March 9, 1998)

Sonographic/Radiographic Report: ACCUVISION DIAGNOSTIC CENTER INC. Name: Sing Kio, Date: 03—09-1998. File No.: 980645. Sonographic/Radiographic Report: Chest X-Ray: Fibrohazed infiltrates noted in both upper lung fields. Rest of the lungs are clear. Hear and the rest of the chest findings are unremarkable. Impression: MINIMAL: PTB. BOTH UPPER LOBES, ACTIVITY UNDETERMINED.

By: Ma. Teresa D. Fontillas, M.D.

My Secret Medicine

Aside from the Tian Xian Liquid, I also used my very own secret medicine. this medicine can't be bought anywhere. You can't ask your friends to look for it. We need to depend on ourselves in order to use this secret medicine. I know everybody is interested to know my secret medicine.

- ◆ Strong Determination
- ◆ Optimistic
- ◆ Courageous Spirit
- ◆ Don't Worry Too Much
- ◆ Don't Be Afraid

This secret that you've hear. is very easy for some of you. But it is hard to apply it in the lives of the cancer patients. We know that in our environment, we have a lot of viruses. But thankfully, our body has antibodies which deals with these viruses. When we are healthy, our antibodies are strong. thus virus can't enter our body. But, when we have a lot of work, or we are hyper-tense, fatigued, stressed-out, our antibody will get low, thus our body becomes vulnerable to viruses.

Thus if a cancer patient is not tense and not nervous, he'll be able to maintain his antibodies. Afterwards, when we drink the medicine, the antibodies will be able to work together with the medicine. On the other hand, if a cancer patient is tensed, scared or afraid, he'll be weak and the medicine won't have any effect on him. This is the primary reason why some of the cancer patients doesn't get cured by Tian Xian Liquid.

Comment by the International Distribution Manager to Mr. Sing Kio's testimony:

I want to comment on the testimony of Mr. Sing Kio. There are some things I would like to bring to everyone's attention. This medicine (Tian Xian Liquid) is most effective when used together with western medicine. Mr. Sing Kio said that he didn't use any western practice (i.e. surgery, chemo), I consider him as "lucky" It is not safe to say that we should only depend on the Tian Xian Liquid, the result will be at its best.

TRIUMPH OVER BREAST CANCER

I REGAIN MY HEALTH BECAUSE OF CHINA NO. 1 TIAN
XIAN LIQUID.
Wang Mi Yun (Aged 41, housewife, Malaysia)

IN LATE 1996, I went for an x-ray examination when I felt pain in my breast.. The doctor said it was a tumor and I should be given special attention. As time went on, the pain increased and the lump on my left breast grew surprisingly fast. When I went to the hospital again, it turned out to be a breast cancer.

I followed the doctor's instruction and had surgery, chemotherapy and radiotherapy. I suffered from diarrhea, vomiting, loss of appetite, loss of weight, and loss of hair. In March of 1997, a doctor friend of my husband learned about China No. 1 Tian Xian Liquid from the Internet and recommended it to us.

I started using it immediately. After three months, an examination of the surgery proved successful for the lymph lump under the armpit had disappeared.

The use of China No. 1 Tian Xian Liquid relieved one from the side-effects of chemotherapy and radiotherapy. I regained my appetite and I felt more energetic than ever before. The most fascinating was the rapid growth of my hair.

Now I go to the hospital for quarterly examination and everything is normal. I finally realized the value of health. I always thank China No. 1 Tian Xian Liquid.

To prevent the recurrence, I still use 20ml a day.

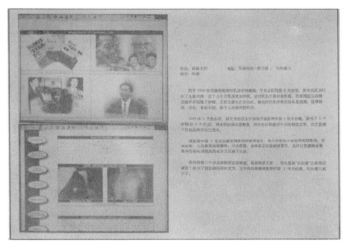

Their doctor friend learns about China No. 1 Tian Xian Liquid from the Internet and introduced it to Ms. Wang.

Triumph Over Breast Cancer

When my doctor said,
'can you accept the fact that you will die?'
My will to combat cancer was heightened
Oohara Mitsuko (Aged 43, housewife, Tottori, Japan)

It was in May when a 5cm tumor in my left breast cancer was discovered. Surgery was performed and chemotherapy followed in three months.

I survived because I learned about China No. 1 Tian Xian Liquid when I was hospitalized. I made a quick decision to use it in mid June. I immediately felt that the side effects of the chemotherapy were eased out.

In addition, I regained my appetite and the number of white blood cells dramatically decreased. The doctors and nurses, who did not know about the liquid were amazed at my improvement. I continue to use China No. 1 Tian Xian Liquid. I will never forget what my doctor said. "other patients of your age and condition died in two months, just get yourself ready...."

Although the doctor never asked me it I could accept death but his clear message only encouraged me to fight harder. I should have thanked him for that.

I think the most important part of my recovery was China No. 1 Tian Xian Liquid. After using it for two years, there was no spread or metastasis. I believe that I must keep on using it. I've taken up my housework. I go out with my family and I enjoy shopping again.

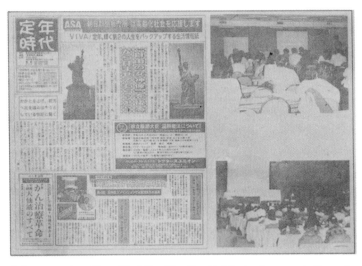

Information about China No. 1 Tian Xian Liquid did not only appear in the media but also in seminars, exhibits and conventions

Triumph Over Breast Cancer

Thanks to China No. 1 Tian Xian Liquid, I can still go to work although I'm afflicted by cancer.
Goto Satsuki (Aged 40, Tokushima, Japan)

When I was diagnosed with breast cancer three years ago, I had surgery immediately. The tumor was 1.5cm and the doctor told me not to worry because it was only in the preliminary stage. However, a later examination showed that it has already spread to my bone tissue. Further diagnosis concluded that I only have one to two years to live.

I did not want to be defeated by cancer after going home, so I continue working. My husband kept looking for a medication that can cure my disease and accompanied me to receive treatments. One day, a Chinese friend brought me some China No. 1 Tian Xian Liquid. After using it for few days, my fatigue was relieved and my energy levels increased. Since then, I have used it everyday. Although cancer cells still remain in my body, it has been three years now and there was no sign of transfer or spreading.

TRIUMPH OVER UTERUS CANCER

I SEE THE TUMOR GETTING SMALLER AND SMALLER
Chen Qing Yun (Aged 48, Guangdong, China)

I CAME from a poor family and needed to work. One day, I felt a severe pain so I went to the hospital. It was so painful that I could not even sit and there was a profuse discharge.

The examination showed that there was a 10cm tumor in the uterus and it was terminal. The doctor said surgery was unavoidable but the

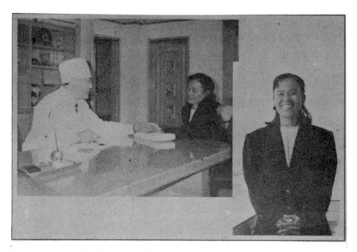

After consulting Mr. Wang, Ms. Chen survives from terminal cancer after using China No. 1 Tian Xian Liquid.

recovery rate was minimal. Finally, I decided to go through surgery even though the pain was severe. I held on to life desperately.

Friends heard about China No. 1 Tian Xian Liquid from the news and its results had been confirmed by clinical tests in hospitals throughout the country. One of my friends had tried it and the results were good. So I began using it too. In about two weeks, the bleeding stopped. One month later, pain had diminished enough that I could afford to sit down.

I got China No. 1 Tian Xian Liquid from the Guangzhou Worker's Hospital. I started using it since March of 1993. In March of 1997, an examination showed that the tumor had reduced to 6cm diameter and now it is down to 3cm diameter. It is progressively getting smaller. After consulting with Mr. Wang, my condition turned out to be good enough for me to go back to work.

Triumph Over Uterus Cancer

IT DOES DECREASE.
Lau Siu Ying (Aged 65, HK)

I WAS diagnosed with a muscle tumor in 1996. Part of my uterus and ovary were removed. To prevent the recurrence, I received radiotherapy afterwards. Cancer cells were discovered again in my uterus in spring of 1997. Further examinations showed that cancer cells had transferred to my chest and brain. It was traumatic! Even after an extensive treatment at the hospital, worst condition persisted.

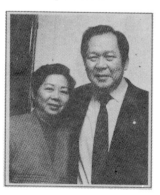

Ms. Lau and her husband using China No. 1 Tian Xian Liquid and capsule to prevent recurrence.

197

The response from the hospital was disappointing. They did not know what to do as surgery was not possible. They suggested more radiotherapy and chemotherapy. I declined because I knew they wouldn't work.

In June, my brother met with Mr. Wang, and he told me to try China No. 1 Tian Xian Liquid. I was excited after hearing that Mr. Wang understood my condition and had advised me to use the liquid and capsule for six months.

Not long after using it, I regained my lost appetite and my condition improved. It's just been six months, nobody now would believe that I suffered from cancer. The doctors could not believe that I miraculously recovered. Then a monthly follow-up examination showed that the new tumor was almost gone and the tumor in my uterus also disappeared.

TRIUMPH OVER UTERUS CANCER

WESTERN MEDICINE ALONE CANNOT CURE ME
Seng Wu Mei (Aged 69, Guangdong, China)

I AM a senior nurse. I had some uterus problems due to menopause in 1990 but I kept on working. However, in August I was diagnosed with uterus cancer.

The tumor was about 9cm diameter and it was in stage 4. I kept hoping that surgery could remove the affected area. After the surgery, I suffered from the horrible side effects of chemotherapy. Two years later, the cancer had transferred to my liver and spleen and the tumor in the uterus recurred.

Even if I had much confidence in Western medicine, I had also learned about China No. 1 Tian Xian Liquid from my patients. I did not believe in it despite a patient's testimony.

Not long after trying it, I felt the effect of the medication. The human body is amazing for it can feel the effect of the medication.

After months of using it, I was released from the side effects of chemotherapy and my body recovered. After applying the liquid and capsule, I was well enough to go back to work.

So I stopped chemotherapy and kept using China No. 1 Tian Xian Liquid and China No. 1 Tian Xian Capsule. It has been ten years now that the uterus cancer has been cured and I am healthier than ever before.

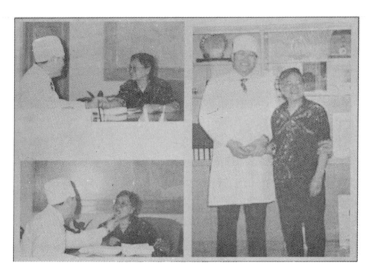

Nurse Zeng during a consultation with Mr. Wang.

TRIUMPH OVER NASOHARYNGEAL PASSAGES CANCER

I AM STILL ALIVE EVEN IF THE SURVIVAL RATE IS
ONLY 15%

Oliver G. Bass (Aged 58, securities company owner,
San Francisco, USA)

"YOU SUFFER from nasopharyngeal passages cancer,' my doctor said.

It was unexpected and I was shocked. I went to the hospital for check up of a cold and it turned out to be cancer.

I pay great attention to my health. I never drink nor smoke. How could I suffer from nasopharyngeal passages cancer? Why did it come so fiercely? It was terminal that even surgery could not help.

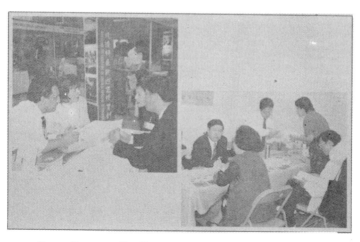

Cancer Seminar in San Francisco attracted much public attentio

It had already spread to the brain and surgery won't help.

I suffered from severe headaches due to the transfer of cancer cells.

Not long after I developed a hearing problem. The doctor said radiation therapy would be the most effective method but the survival rate was only 15%. I did not have any other choice.

The side effects of radiation therapy are exceptionally difficult (vomiting, oral cavity inflammation, sore throat). Even drinking could have killed me. I cannot forget the feeling of being mute.

Then I learned about China No. 1 Tian Xian Liquid from the news and I tried it. The hospital allowed me to go home after radiotherapy of my first stage of cancer. I took six bottles a day and after only two weeks, I could go shopping, read newspapers and watch TV. My skin then was darkened by the radiation but regained its original complexion and further examinations showed that all cancer cells had disappeared.

Triumph Over Nasoharyngeal Passages Cancer

I relied only on China No. 1 Tian Xian Liquid even after going through chemotherapy
Zhou Yu Zen (Aged 58, carpenter, Taichung, Taiwan)

In February of 1997, I went to the hospital for an examination of a swollen lymph gland. The result indicated that I am suffering from nasopharyngeal passages cancer.

The doctor said that concentrated radiotherapy from four to five times can cure me within two months so I accepted the arrangement. The treatment caused great pain in my nose with a dry throat. I could not sleep, my overall condition was getting worse. I lost 10 kg from my original weight!

Then I had chemotherapy a 500cc injection in my body. I felt weakened. The four month treatment resulted in more anxiety.

After learning of the effect of China No. 1 Tian Xian Liquid from my friend, I immediately went to Hong Kong to buy it. I did not know that it was available in Taiwan.

Two months after using it together with chemotherapy, my body recovered exceptionally well. After completing chemotherapy, I relied only on China No. 1 Tian Xian Liquid.

One year after the treatment, an examination showed that it was completely gone. The doctor advised me to continue using China No. 1 Tian Xian Liquid.

Triumph Over Lymph Cancer

I believe in Chinese Medicine
Wang Zin Yuan (Aged 44, designer, Guangdong, China)

I HAD stomach problem for about six months and I knew that it wasn't good. I thought I had a liver problem. My friend thought it was gall bladder problem. I even felt severe pain in the kidney and sometimes in the back. I went to the hospital for detailed examination.

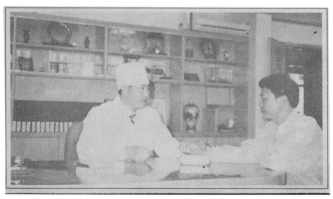

Mr. Wang regained his health because of his faith in China No. 1 Tian Xian Liquid.

The result showed a chronic gall bladder inflammation and a 2.5 x 2cm ulcer in the liver. A CT scan indicated that it was blood vessel cancer. The doctor decided to remove the tumor before confirming whether it was benign or malignant. The surgery on April 12 confirmed the presence of lymph cancer. Chemotherapy and radiotherapy followed and their side effects affected my appetite and experienced loss of hair.

I was so depressed. I would try anything to survive. Then my boss told me about China No.1 Tian Xian Liquid and I tried it without thinking. I learned of its effects from books and magazines.

Even the doctors said that Chinese medicine could not help but I still believed that it could. After using it, I regained my lost appetite and grew my hair. Although sometimes the wound could cause pain, I don't need to worry about cancer now.

Triumph Over Lymph Cancer

For the sake of my wife and myself,
I shall never surrender
Wang Qing Biao (Aged 37, food processing,
Yuehlin, Taiwan)

In April of 1997, lumps were found in my throat and armpit. The local hospital diagnosed them as chronic inflammation. I thought it was nothing but six months later more lumps were found in the lymph throughout my body. I kept losing weight so I went to the hospital in Taipei for further examination.

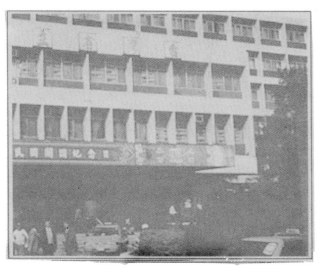

Chemotherapy and China No. 1 Tian Xian Liquid helped me recover from cancer.

The diagnosis showed that it was lymph cancer stage four. I could not believe it after hearing the truth. I did not know what to do next. Fortunately, my wife kept encouraging me and I tried chemotherapy which resulted in vomiting, uneasiness and loss of hair. I was in great pain.

I suffered a lot from the side effects. A marrow examination showed that cancer was already inside. I felt hopeless.

A co-worker brought me some China No. 1 Tian Xian Liquid. I tried it together with the chemotherapy. In May and July of 1998 after the examinations, the doctors told me that I was very lucky and there were almost no cancer cells in the marrow. They thought it was the work of chemotherapy but I believe it was China No. 1 Tian Xian Liquid.

Now the cancer cells are gone. The doctor told me that rate of lymph cancer to recur is very high so I continue to use China No. 1 Tian Xian Liquid and China No. 1 Tian Xian Capsule. I am very glad to have regained my health. Thanks to my wife and to China No. 1 Tian Xian Liquid.

Triumph Over Lymph Cancer

Recovered quickly from Symptoms
Kong Chi Keung (Aged 77, HK)

In the spring, I suddenly lost my consciousness. I was very strong so it was really surprising. It turned out to be the result of a brain tumor. My age and condition made surgery impossible. I was hospitalized after examining that water has accumulated in my heart and lungs I was

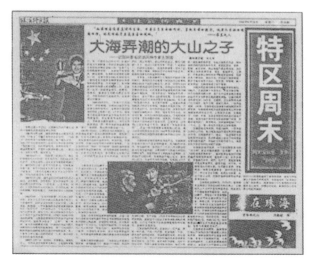

My friend who introduced me to China No. 1 Tian Xian Liquid gave me much hope.

diagnosed with lymph cancer. The doctor told me that my chances of survival was less than 20% even with radiotherapy and chemotherapy were applied.

The condition worsened and I lost a lot of body weight. That autumn, a friend of mine told me about the effects of China No. 1 Tian Xian Liquid. I bought some after learning more about it. After using it for two months, I regained my lost weight, I used it secretly together with chemotherapy.

Loss of appetite and hair is normal result of chemotherapy but I had neither not even vomiting.

I had worked in a weaving factory and gas station. The doctor said that the latter might have contributed to my disease. But as a strong 70-year old, I did not agree with his opinion.

In December, an examination indicated that the lymph cancer had reduced incredibly and my condition improved to the extent that I could work already. When my condition has stabilized, I left the hospital immediately. I continued to use China No. 1 Tian Xian suppository. I am very glad that I survived.

Triumph Over Lymph Cancer

It's true! China No. 1 Tian Xian Liquid made
the tumor smaller
Ma Mi Yu (Aged 46, housewife, Bangkok, Thailand)

I WENT to the hospital for a throat problem. The doctor said it was just minor inflammation and he gave me some antibiotics. However, the problem did not get solved. Since I needed to take care of my children, I just had to live with it.

In September of 1995, my neck began itching. I scraped it and began bleeding uncontrollably. I was rushed to the hospital and lymph cancer was discovered. Surgery was advised in the following next month to

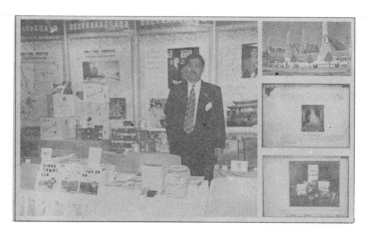

Information on China No. 1 Tian Xian Liquid is available on the internet in Chinese, English, Japanese, Spanish, German, French, Hindi, Korean and Arabic (see http://www.cancerherbal.com)

remove two lymph tumors in three areas. But the doctor had to leave one of them as it was very close to the main artery.

Fortunately, my husband is hardworking and we don't have any financial problem. We could afford to use Chinese medicine together with chemotherapy. We learned about China No. 1 Tian Xian Liquid in the Internet so we went to a drugstore in Bangkok to buy some. Although I recovered a bit after using it, the pain has increased sharply. My condition got worse and I could still feel the depression.

One day, I read a news report from Hong Kong paper I thought to my self, 'was I deceived?' After comparing the pictures in the papers with China No. 1 Tian Xian Liquid I was using, I found out the truth I was cheated. According to the news, there are so many counterfeits. I must say that only authentic products have real effects. After learning the telephone number of the global agent, we immediately ordered it from Hong Kong. When it arrived, I checked it with the pictures in the papers. It was the real thing.

Certainly, the effect of the authentic product was real. My pain disappeared in a month. After six months, the tumor was much smaller. Maybe it is the work of both chemotherapy and China No.1 Tian Xian Liquid.

Just when I thought I could stop using it and rely merely on chemotherapy, I immediately lost my energy. My condition went downhill and the pain returned. Examinations showed that the tumor grew back so I immediately started to use China No. 1 Tian Xian Liquid again. Now, I will never stop using it until I am sure that my tumor is completely gone.

Now I principally use China No. 1 Tian Xian Liquid and the capsule and suppository according to my needs. The lymph tumor reduced in size to the point that I can hardly feel it.

TRIUMPH OVER CANCER

DUE TO MARROW CANCER, I HAVE LESS THAN THREE
MONTHS TO LIVE.
Bagesu Kerian (Aged 57, professor of South Africa
University, South Africa)

WHEN A marrow tumor was discovered by Dr. Kojjya Portgay, I thought that advanced medical treatment can cure me. In April of 1995, an examination showed that it has recurred.

'Sorry, it has already spread to your hand, you have only three months.'

Even though I had accepted that I might die soon, I could not stand

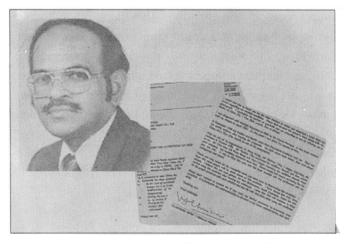

Professor Bagesu was pronounced to live less than 3 months.

by hopelessly and fail my family. I gave up everything and began packing everything. In July, I received a letter from my brother who was working at the Indian Embassy. He told me about China No. 1 Tian Xian Liquid. He insisted that I try it. I did not have much faith in it but I tried it because I wanted to stay longer with my family. A miracle came after using it in just two months. I was recovering and later examination even surprised Dr. Kojjya. In May of 1997, an examination showed no sign of cancer cells. Periodic blood and marrow tests show everything is normal.

A miracle happened to me. I survived and I am cured. I believe other people can make it, too. Never give up! Trust China No. 1 Tian Xian Liquid and its powers!

Triumph Over Cancers

I subscribe directly from Hong Kong and finally
I saw the truth about urethra cancer
Eto Koji (Aged 40, office clerk, Nagoya, Japan)

In August 6 of 1997, I was hospitalized because of blood in my urine. In February, I went to a local hospital but they found nothing and I was discharged after three weeks of hospitalization. To find out the truth, I went back to the same hospital again and received different examinations but no medications were given.

Further examinations on August 20 showed that there were three tumors in my urethra. Surgery was necessary to remove the urethra and the left kidney. Subsequent examinations proved that it was malignant tumor.

My family kept searching for new medicines and treatments. From the Internet, they learned about China No. 1 Tian Xian Liquid and they ordered it from Hong Kong. They brought the liquid and the capsule to the hospital. On September 8, I began with one capsule and four bottles per day. In about one week's time, the same examinations showed that the tumors in the urethra were gone. So the doctor postponed the surgery after 2 weeks. I recovered very well after the surgery. So I left the hospital on January 22. Now, I live happily everyday and I still use China No. 1 Tian Xian Liquid at a reduced dosage.

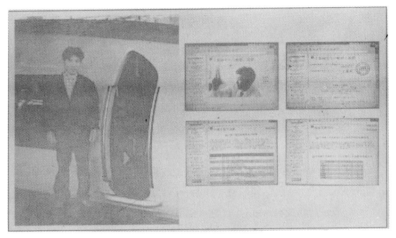

Mr. Eto learned about China No. 1 Tian Xian Liquid from the Internet.

TRIUMPH OVER CANCERS

JOY TO SEE NEW LIFE-ORAL CAVITY CANCER
Bing Guang (Aged 36, teacher, Hsinchu, Taiwan)

I AM so happy because ·I am getting married and I want to build a home of my own.

In August of 1998, I felt severe pain on my tongue so I went to the hospital. The result showed that it was preliminary stage of oral cavity cancer and half of my tongue needed to be removed! Both my wife and I could not accept this because I was going to be a father. Due to my wife's support and encouragement from my friends, I decided to fight against cancer.

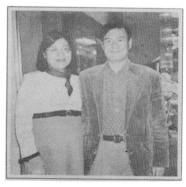

For the sake of my baby, I overcame cancer with the love and support of my wife.

To overcome cancer, I devoted myself learning the truth about the disease. Some information was given by my relatives. It seemed that surgery was inevitable. I began using China No. 1 Tian Xian Liquid as a supplement ten days before the surgery. I looked at my tongue in front of the mirror everyday to measure any change because I was expecting a miracle from China No.1 Tian Xian Liquid.

The miracle came before the surgery! A CT scan before the surgery showed that the tumor had reduced in size which means that they would only cut off a small part of my tongue.

The doctor told me that it would not effect my speech or eating and those facts comforted me a lot.

The post-surgery examinations showed that there was no sign of transfer or expansion. No chemotherapy or radiotherapy was needed. Regular examination and dietary care were necessary. It must be the mercy of God. I experienced the darkness of life and I realized the joy of life in those few months.

It was a test of my chastity. I will never forget that China No. 1 Tian Xian Liquid is my savior. I still use it everyday. I also change my diet according to the information given by the global agent, China Japan Feida Union Co., Ltd.

I am very confident now and I am enjoying my role as a father. Of course, the experience made me realize the importance of health.

No matter what your plan is, if you don't have good health, everything will end up to nothing. For my baby, I am sure that I will give him a healthier life.

Finally, I must thank my wife who has always been with me and of course, China No. 1 Tian Xian Liquid which has saved my life.

Combined use of China No. 1 Tian Xian Liquid with chemotherapy, no metastatic effect and I got better from my pharynx cancer
Tanaka Masatoshi (Aged 64, merchant, Saga, Japan)

In February of 1996, I was hospitalized and diagnosed with pharynx cancer at a local hospital. Chemotherapy was performed followed by surgery.

The surgery went well. I went home in April. Just as I could enjoy my new life I received horrible news. An examination showed recurrence of cancer. Doctors told me that only radiotherapy could help.

A neighbor introduced China No. 1 Tian Xian Liquid to me. He had been cured by it. So I used it while receiving chemotherapy. I took six vials a day for three months. The pain stopped and the tumor disappeared. The doctor said that there was no sign of metastasis. I am better and stronger now, I still use China No. 1 Tian Xian Liquid everyday.

Appendix-About the International Rehabilitation of Cancer Association

AN ORGANIZATION WHICH SUPPORTS PATIENTS WHO COMBAT CANCER WORLDWIDE

THE ASSOCIATION is based in Hong Kong and headed by Mr. Wang Zhen-Guo. It is an organization that supports patients combating cancer worldwide. As the Director of the association and researcher of the National Health Department, I have established a base in Hong Kong with the support of the China Japan Feida Union Co., Ltd.

Because there are about 40 million people who suffer from cancer, the association is engaged in all kinds of activities aimed at eradicating cancer from this world. We provide free treatment and information to patients in poor countries of South East Asia.

To participate in all kinds of international cancer conventions, I deliver lectures and prepare seminars. So far, we have organized over 10 lectures and seminars in Japan.

The association will exhaust all efforts to eradicate cancer from this world and to organize support activities to help cancer patients worldwide.

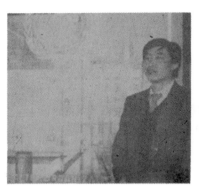
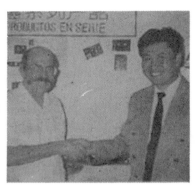

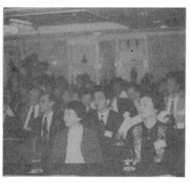
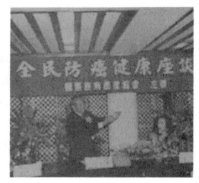

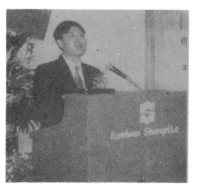
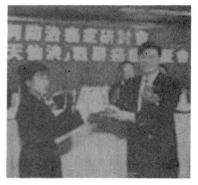

EPILOGUE

NEVER SURRENDER TO CANCER

FOR THOSE who have overcome cancer, I can see how much they have to go through. I think they must have something in common: courage and love of their families.

When they have courage to overcome cancer they must have obtained the love from their families. They should know that they have to survive and to do something for them. When their families have given them greatest support, that is the very motivation which enabled them to overcome cancer.

Cancer is a dreadful disease but we should not give up. You must believe that you can cure cancer with family support and encouragement.

The content of this book will make you fully understand the effect of China No. 1 Tian Xian Liquid. But I don't think that is the end. Cancer patients have increased every day so that we have to improve our medication to cure the dreadful disease.

Therefore, I strongly hope that Western and Chinese medicines will give up discriminating each other. The attitude to prevent and cure cancer should be the common objective of both sides. Our task means that we should try everything within our capabilities.

Absolutely the best is that cancer cells are not even found inside your body. Unfortunately, if you become a cancer patient one-day, please do not be frightened because cancer is curable. So never give up.

I am sure that there are 5-6 kindsd of counterfeits that have been found in Hong Kong, Taiwan and Japan. Counterfeits are incredible, they use the same packaging but only contained syrup. Even if we opened the formula to the public, the products will never be the same because of the difference in processing.

Counterfeits are openly displayed in drugstores in Hong Kong and Taiwan, sometimes even licensed pharmacists and doctors join the line. So you must be very careful.

China No. 1 Tian Xian Liquid has been launched in Japan for several years already. Thanks to the media, the cancer buster China No. 1 Tian Xian Liquid and its amazing effects improved cancer treatment. Currently there are about 20,000 individuals who take China No. 1 Tian Xian Liquid in Japan alone.

I have never dreamt that China No. 1 Tian Xian Liquid which was born in Changbai Mountain would gain worldwide popularity. It proved that my faith in Chinese medicine to cure cancer was right. I will continue my work to save more cancer patients. I will let the public know more about the Tian Xian Liquid. I will teach them to distinguish the fake from the authentic ones and thereby set up several branches worldwide.

This is the third book I have published in Japan. After I have set up the inquiry service in Japan -WANG Zhen-Guo Office- Japan Branch, I was able to collect much information and made the publication possible. I have spent great effort and time on this book and I believe that there is a lot of information to benefit from.

My gratitude to the many people who have given me encouragement and assistance in completing this book especially the grammarians, translators, researchers and those who documented the materials and the China-Japan Feida Union Co., Ltd.

Finally, my deep gratitude to my wife.

WANG Zhen-Guo
20 March 1999 at Zhuhai

ABOUT THE AUTHOR

MR. WANG Zhen-Guo was born in 1954 in Tonghua City, Jilin, China. He graduated from the Tonghua City Sanitation School (medical school) in 1975. He developed China No. 1 Tian Xian Pill in 1983 which was later approved by the government of China to be an effective anti cancer medication in 1988. Then he continued with the development of the more effective China No. 1 Tian Xian Liquid. In 1989, his achievements were recognized when he received the Best Personal Achievement Award in 1989 and the Royal Medal in Belgium.

He is now a researcher of the National Health Department, supervisor at the International Rehabilitation of Cancer, Director of the Jilin Anti Cancer Association, Changbai Mountain Pharmacology Research Institute, Deputy Director of the China Anti Cancer foundation and Deputy Director of the Jilin Anti Cancer Association.

His publications are chiefly published in China and subsequently in Japan, Hong Kong, Taiwan, the Philippines and Malaysia. He has published a great number of research papers.

NOTES

NOTES

NOTES

_____

_____

_____

_____

_____

_____

_____

_____

_____

_____

_____

_____

_____

_____

_____

_____

_____

_____

_____

_____

_____

_____

_____

_____